I0110462

A BRUTAL DISEASE

A BRUTAL DISEASE

Motor Neuron Disease during
the Pandemic

Manzoor G K Ishani

THE CHOIR PRESS

Copyright © 2025 Manzoor G K Ishani

All rights reserved. No part of this publication may be reproduced or
transmitted in any form or by any means, electronic or mechanical
including photocopying, recording or any information storage or
retrieval system, without prior permission in writing from the publishers.

The right of Manzoor G K Ishani to be identified as the author of this
work has been asserted by him in accordance with the Copyright,
Designs and Patents act 1988

First published in the United Kingdom in 2025 by

The Choir Press

ISBN 978-1-78963-525-6

For Marilyn, of course.

No spring, nor summer beauty hath such grace
As I have seen in one autumnal face.

John Donne

Preface

This is a story about Marilyn, my wife of more than fifty three years, who was struck down with motor neuron disease. It is about me, who perforce became her sole life support, and it's about the challenges we faced. It is about the storm which raged within her as she struggled with her terminal illness, and how Brexit and COVID left us floundering in virtually total isolation.

The first part of this book seeks to explain the nature of Marilyn's illness and how the two of us tried to deal with the physical, emotional and medical effect it had on us. The second part is more about me, the challenges I faced during the pandemic that was COVID-19 and its consequences for me. The rest tells of my attempt to overcome the emotional turmoil that was beginning to overwhelm me after Marilyn died, and buried within it is an account of the trials and tribulations that Marilyn had to endure.

By the way, don't go checking any statistics you may come across too carefully, as I am not a details person. Though I may have some pretensions to literacy, I'm wholly innumerate. 'Fiscal rectitude' sounds to me like a cure for haemorrhoids, 'stagflation' sounds like a sport played at Balmoral and 'quantitative easing' sounds like the consequence of taking an enema. I tend to prize presentation and bluff over hard graft, and usually rely on a silk square in my top pocket, a well-knotted tie and polished shoes to get me over the line in tight situations – can't think why. In the words of Edward Gibbon, 'style is the image of character'.

Although I don't have a therapist, you will see references to 'my therapist' because it sounds cool. I do, however, have a remarkable GP[1] who was always at hand to lend support.

Our elder son Rafik proved to be a rock in times of need providing much needed support on the 'phone' in moments of deep crisis and Zahir his younger brother also helped with sourcing much need equipment. Sadly our quarantine prevented them from doing more

The names of characters in this chronicle have been changed to protect the innocent, although they are far from innocent.

My apologies, dear reader, that this is not a bodice-ripping yarn; it does, however, have its moments.

If you are flicking through the pages in 'a good bookshop somewhere near you', wondering whether to buy it, I would urge you to buy two copies: one for your library at home, and one for the library on your yacht.

---

[1] Dr Richard Draper MRCGP, a physician who possesses the rare skill of being ever mindful of the need to treat the patient as well as the illness.

THE CHALLENGE

There's no shame in fear ... what matters is how we face it.

George RR Martin

Death comes to us all ...

It all started in 2019, on a day in the first week of May, when, in conversation with Marilyn, I noticed she was slurring some of her words. She found it difficult to pronounce the letters 's', 'x' and 'z' succinctly. She saw her GP, who took her blood pressure, which showed a reading of 149/94. He gave her an aspirin and arranged for her to be seen at A&E at Epsom General Hospital as a matter of urgency.

She was seen by a doctor immediately and, after some tests, he came to a possible diagnosis of a stroke. Marilyn was admitted as an inpatient and was subjected to further tests over the following three days. The results defeated the diagnosis of a stroke and she was referred to a neurologist, who, following a general examination, saw her the following week for further tests as an outpatient.

Of all the tests and examinations, the most exacting was what came to be known to us as the 'needle test'. This involved Marilyn lying perfectly still while a consultant inserted into her various muscles no fewer than twelve

1

needles, each of which was attached by a thin wire to a monitor through which an electrical current was passed, to see how (if at all) each muscle reacted to the current. The pain was perceived to be so intense that they tried to prevent my being present, lest I should try to intervene to prevent the test from continuing (as was their experience in the past with others). I remained in the room.

The Disease

The neurologist, in the presence of a nurse (presumably in anticipation of a possible emotional meltdown by one or both of us), informed us of the diagnosis: motor neuron disease. The prognosis was six to nine months. There was no cure.

At the time we, like most, were unaware of motor neuron disease. Marilyn had assumed that the worst diagnosis would be that of dysarthria, which results from weak neck muscles, rendering speech difficult but for which there is the prospect of ameliorating the symptoms with speech therapy. It was much worse; dysarthria was to be only one of many symptoms which would manifest themselves over time.

There were no histrionics and no emotional meltdown; we were in a state of deep shock and speechless. The realisation at that moment that I was living and that she was dying tore me apart. As I said to the GP later that day, 'It should have been *me*.'

Motor neuron disease (MND) is a rare condition which affects the brain and the nervous system. It causes muscular weakness which gets worse over time. There is no cure for

MND, which can significantly shorten life expectancy; it is cruel, it is brutal and it is fatal.

The disease affects signals transmitted by the brain to the muscles via the nervous system. It is a rapidly progressive disease which is caused by a problem with brain cells and nerves called motor neurons and affects the spinal cord. It attacks the nerves that control movement so muscles refuse to work. It can leave people locked in a failing body, unable to move and eventually to breathe. It's not known why this happens. The symptoms vary from one patient to another. It mainly affects people in their sixties and seventies.

In Marilyn's case the disease severely affected her ability to speak, to move limbs, swallow, sniff, cough, shed tears, and control the flow of saliva; within a few weeks she was unable to communicate by spoken word. Breathing became increasingly difficult and finally impossible. Yet, with an IQ of 142, Marilyn's brain remained razor-sharp right to the very end.

A sense of urgency compelled us to discuss matters of a practical nature, in terms of both coping with the disease and the daily grind of living. In the case of the former, she had to choose between fighting the disease and adopting an attitude which would enable her to deal with whatever symptoms the MND would bring. It took no discussion. True to her character, she had already settled on a positive attitude. However, this, she said, was conditional; she didn't want to know how the disease might progress, its symptoms etc. She would tackle them as and when they manifested themselves. It was preferable, she said, to dwelling on what was reasonably foreseeable. I felt the same way, but in my case I had to know and to anticipate what was likely to happen.

My research into the disease, its symptoms and the manner of its progression, horrified me.

What is known about MND is infinitesimal compared to how much is not known. Our knowledge of the universe and outer space is humongous in comparison to what is known about MND. Just as, prior to the exploration of space, its vastness was unknown, so today is the vastness of the unknown of what causes and what might cure MND.

What defeats the acquisition of our knowledge of this disease is its uber rarity. It is estimated that 0.01% of the population are affected by this disease: that is to say roughly 7,000 people out of a population of 70 million people, and they are spread out over an area of 95,000 square miles. This is insufficient to provide the critical mass needed for effective investigation, research and discovery of a possible cure.

As Dr Robin Howard remarked, 'In my forty years of medical practice concerned with this disease, I know less today than I did yesterday. That is to say that it is so rare and its symptoms so varied in each case that they defy any coherent theory of its cause and therefore obstruct the discovery of a possible cure. Important research is being done, but we are a long way off finding a cure.'

I consoled myself with the knowledge that soon Marilyn would be cared for by specialists, nurses and carers. Marilyn told me she wanted to die at home and I readily agreed, switching my efforts to arranging domiciliary care and putting my mind to the practical realities and difficulties which that entailed.

Little did I know at the time that no such support would be available. In May 2022, the Association of Directors of

Adult Social Services announced that the number of adults waiting for care in England had risen to more than half a million. Its president, Sarah McClinton, said it was having 'a devastating impact on people's lives'. Since the spring of 2021 there had been a sevenfold increase in hours that could not be delivered because of a shortage of care workers. We were soon to be on our own for the duration.

I set about converting our ground floor into a mini hospital ward, moving furniture, removing doors and catering for the possible conversion of a room into an intensive care unit.

Physical Care

We faced our first challenge within a few weeks: Brexit, and its consequences for us. The Spanish cleaners fled back to Spain and I was left with no help, so to my daily tasks of shopping and cooking were added washing, ironing, cleaning etc.: essentially those of a full-time housekeeper. I tried desperately to manage the house with the silent efficiency of a Silver Ghost.

It wasn't long before Marilyn began to find it increasingly difficult to manage for herself. Attending to personal hygiene, dressing, eating and drinking became a herculean task for her. We were determined that she should be as independent as possible and for as long as possible. I replaced her wardrobe with 'user-friendly' garments such as linen smocks which she could throw over her head. I sought out special scissors and other aids to help her undertake daily tasks, like buttoning a blouse, operating the zip on her house gown etc. They very soon became redundant. Thank heavens for the much-maligned 'next-day delivery' services (until the significant COVID clampdown), and for online banking; it wasn't long before our credit cards had reached their limits.

Following on the heels of Brexit came COVID-19. The nation was in lockdown. Marilyn, being severely vulnerable, was placed under quarantine at home and, as her carer, so was I. By now she had little or no resistance to infection. Given that she was unable to cough, sneeze or sniff, a simple cold would have caused her unimaginable grief.

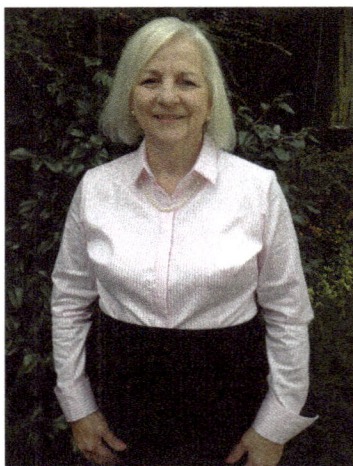

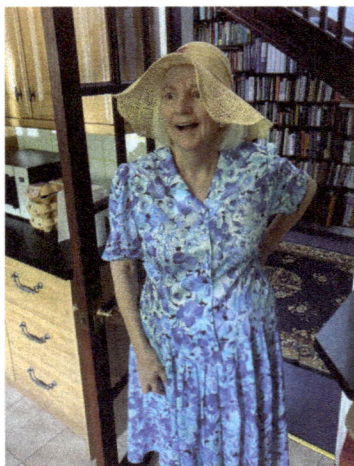

Before MND   *Some months later*
                          (early stages of decline)

All help and support which had so far been available or in the pipeline vanished overnight. Henceforth a strict protocol was enforced. This may seem harsh in hindsight, but, although a member of the medical profession, whatever their métier, may have tested negative, they were being exposed to COVID on a daily basis. They may not have exhibited the symptoms of COVID, but they may have been carriers. The safest course of action to protect Marilyn from being exposed to the disease was to allow no one to cross the threshold, whatever their status, function or profession, though relatively little help was available in any case. Furthermore, I was soon to discover that there was now no readily available ambulance/paramedic service.

To my list of extended duties were now added those of clinical nurse, palliative carer and quasi-paramedic (more about this later). With them there also grew the demand on my time, and as a result the day grew longer. During the last one and a half years of Marilyn's life I worked a seventeen-to eighteen-hour day, seldom fewer. Hour by hour, day by day, I was spinning plates, all the while fearful lest one of them should fall crashing to the floor.

Before long, Marilyn began to struggle with swallowing. Breakfast now consisted of very runny scrambled eggs and some orange juice. A miniscule amount was ingested by placing the egg on her tongue on a little plastic pusher (of the type to be found in small ice cream tubs) and easing it down. It was essential that nothing should make its way down her windpipe; given her declining lung capacity, it was likely to cause an infection, which could result in her death. All in all, it would take her half an hour or more to ingest two teaspoons of egg and a few drops of orange juice. In the beginning I cooked soft food, such as fish and chicken, which I liquidised.

I was becoming aware of the need for Marilyn to undergo surgery to accommodate feeding tubes into her stomach by means of percutaneous endoscopic gastrostomy (PEG). A PEG tube was to be threaded through her gut and out through her stomach wall for use to feed her directly into the stomach. It was designed to meet all her nutritional needs.

Given COVID restrictions, how this was to be achieved was a matter of debate. The good Lord smiles on the virtuous; we were blessed with the temporary relaxation of COVID restrictions between COVID 1 and COVID 2 when association amongst individuals was permitted, albeit in limited numbers and restricted to the open air. After some frantic phone calls, an appointment was made for Marilyn to be admitted at the National Hospital for Neurology and Neurosurgery in Queen's Square, London.

The night before her admission, Marilyn was becoming anxious. She scribbled a note to me: *no genl anasthtic* [sic] *afraid I not wake up*. My mantra to all who attended to her was 'What Mrs Ishani wants, Mrs Ishani gets.' So a strong local anaesthetic was administered.

When we arrived we were faced with locked doors, affixed to which was a note with a mobile number. Upon making the call, the door was opened by a nurse and a security guard, to whom I showed a hard copy of the email I had received.

The nurse accompanied us to the fourth floor and, as we approached the ward, it dawned on me that it was no longer possible to wander into a ward. Access was only by means of a swipe card. Accompanied as we were by the nurse, we were given entry and ushered to a waiting room, where we were to wait for four hours before Marilyn's bed became available.

After about two hours I went to the nurses' station to enquire if there was a toilet I could use, only to be informed that toilets were for patients only and that if I wanted to relieve myself I would have to go to outpatients, to be found in the building next door. On my return, muttering, 'When the going gets tough, the toffs get going!' I strode authoritatively past the security guard, brushing him aside with a wave of my hand, and proceeded to the ward. Once on the threshold, I realised that I had no swipe card to gain entry to the ward, and so I knocked on a long glass panel on the door, through which I caught the eye of a nurse who opened the door and let me in.

On my way back to the waiting room I passed a small ward containing four beds. There I saw two men on their hands and knees, sanitising the wheels and frame of a bed and the surrounding floor. I now understood why it had taken four hours to prepare a bed for Marilyn.

I stayed with Marilyn throughout the day, after helping her to unpack, and returned the following morning, adopting the same procedure for gaining entry by striding past the now-familiar security guard and knocking on the glass panel on the door. On the third day the hospital telephoned me to say that they were ready to discharge Marilyn and asked if I would come to collect her. This I did, gaining entry to the ward in the usual manner.

I was met at Marilyn's bedside by a staff nurse who said she was pleased to say that the surgery had been successful, that there were no complications and that it was now possible to discharge Marilyn. What was now required, she said, was to train her carer. 'Where is Mrs Ishani's carer?' she asked, only to be told that she was looking at him. The look of surprise and puzzlement on her face said it all. She told me that she would train me on how to attend to the surgical wound (change the dressings etc.) over the next few days.

She pulled back the bedclothes, stripped off the gauze, dressing, surgical tape etc., and, having done that, to my surprise she then replaced it all. Then she stripped it all off again and asked me to dress the wound in the same way she had.

I had watched her carefully and, with some trepidation, proceeded as shown until I came to the stage where I had to apply the surgical tape. To cut this I did what I have done for most of my life, particularly at Christmas. I moved the surgical tape towards my mouth and, in time-honoured fashion, was about to tear it with my teeth, only to hear the staff nurse shout, 'STOP! Use the scissors. I'm really surprised, given that you are a doctor. You should know better.'

'A doctor?' I queried. 'I'm not a doctor; who told you I am a doctor?'

'The nurses at the desk tell me you are Mrs Ishani's doctor; that's why they have been admitting you and allowing you to stay with her all day. The only people who are allowed in the presence of a patient are the medical staff attending to their patients.'

This is not the first time that I have been mistaken for a doctor. Must be my demeanour.

Now, it so happens that I am pretty useless when it comes to handling sticky tape – all fingers and thumbs, though I did dress the wound and feeding tubes roughly in the manner instructed. True enough, a lot of the tape was, not to put too fine a point on it, untidy and bunched. The nurse looked at me, shook her head and said, 'Well, this is not at all as I showed you, is it?'

An image of Peggy Mount superimposed on that of Hattie Jacques flitted across my mind. I muttered under my breath, 'What I don't need right now is a ticking-off.'

She proceeded to undo everything and asked me to do it again. 'Properly this time, please.'

I made a better job of it the second time around and explained that, in my opinion, the result was not too dissimilar to what she had done.

'Well, it's not quite the same, is it?'

My frustration and exasperation having now got the better of me, I said, 'Looks to me as if everything is in place and secure. Who's the doctor here, anyway?'

If looks could kill. Showering me with thin praise, she muttered, 'Well, OK, I suppose it will get better with practice.'

She now led me to another room to train me in the process of cleaning, preparing and administering the feeding tube and the syringes needed for this, and in the maintenance of the tube and the fixator. The fixator was a mechanism which would allow me to release the tube from its housing, enabling me to turn the tube ever so carefully on a weekly basis, to prevent it from seizing up when tissue grew over it as Marilyn's body naturally tried to heal the incision.

The exact doses and timings were predetermined. This would involve me administering twenty-seven syringes in each twenty-four-hour cycle, and each time the syringes had to be meticulously washed out and sterilised in readiness for the next session, as did various other equipment, such as the ventilator and suction machine.

On the day of Marilyn's discharge the restrictions which applied to COVID 1 were reimposed with the advent of COVID 2. It was a narrow escape and we felt lucky to have got this done.

I breathed a deep sigh of relief and took comfort in knowing that Marilyn could now 'eat and drink'. At this stage the greatest concern was that she should ramp up her weight to the maximum possible, because when eventually her digestive system started failing she would begin to lose weight, and once the weight loss set in there was no possibility of her regaining it.

I now added to my tasks the administration of fibre, protein, water, nutrient supplements and medication by the use of syringes, all the time having to make sure that the right dose was administered at the right time and ensuring that everything was sterilised well in readiness for the next session.

I took Marilyn home and settled her down. The day had gone smoothly. For me it was one of the best days ever; everything went as planned, and Marilyn's equilibrium was not disturbed. We were both relieved. I felt I had achieved something. It felt good. Another battle won. Tomorrow was to be another day … and so it proved to be.

Just after five o'clock in the morning, Marilyn summoned me and indicated that she was in pain. When I took off the bedcovers I saw that not only was her wound weeping but she was bleeding as well. This was something that I had neither expected nor anticipated. There were no paramedics immediately available. I couldn't begin to understand the pain she was in, given that where it was not possible for her to swallow a couple of painkillers.

I left a message for the neurologist's consultant nurse for MND on her mobile. She called me back about an hour later and, after I had explained what had happened, she promised to call me back within ten minutes and arrange a district nurse to visit. She called me back straight away only to inform me that the district nurse was not available, she having been summoned to a Nightingale Hospital: temporary critical care hospitals set up for the pandemic.

It was all hands on deck and, regrettably, there was nobody available to assist.

From my description of what was happening, the consultant nurse had ascertained the nature of the problem: the surgeon may have been a little aggressive, and the fixator had been digging into Marilyn, cutting into the surface of her stomach.

The only option was to take Marilyn to A&E, which in reality was no option at all. I nervously asked if there was anything else that could be done. The consultant nurse said it involved a medical procedure and explained what needed to be done in some detail. She asked if I was willing to try to do it.

I looked at Marilyn and asked her if she was willing to take the risk. The consultant nurse had made it clear that the consequences of my getting it wrong could be that the tube would be released from its housing in the stomach and come away. Marilyn, her eyes now red with fear, indicated that I should go ahead.

That she should have so much confidence in me was the greatest compliment I have ever been paid. It boosted my confidence, and I found myself in a situation where, for once, having found the confidence, I now lacked the competence. I became fearful, a fear within me which is difficult to describe. This, I told myself, is not a movie where a passenger in the pilot's cockpit is guided by Charlton Heston in the control tower into landing the plane with an unconscious pilot slumped over the controls.

The consultant nurse talked me through the procedure again. I followed her instructions through misty eyes as she took me through step by step. All this was done via the telephone, with no access to FaceTime or any visual aid.

As soon as I had finished, my hands started shaking uncontrollably and tears cascaded down my cheeks. I squeezed Marilyn's hand, cleansed the wound, changed the dressing, and the bedding.

As instructed, I watched over the wound for the next few hours to ensure that all was well. Mercifully it was. It was not an experience I would wish on anyone.

From then on, all food and drink – medication, nutrients, supplements, water, protein, fibre etc. – was ingested by Marilyn through the PEG. So, all in all, a good result. Another battle fought well and won.

What will be next? I asked myself.

I knew that the time would come when she would need assistance with her breathing. This would be via a ventilator. To take advantage of the greater relaxation of COVID restrictions, I arranged for Marilyn to go back into hospital to be tested for her respiratory efficiency. She was admitted for two nights and a day whilst they monitored her lung function, breathing pattern and oxygen intake. Upon her discharge from the hospital I was trained on the use, monitoring, cleaning etc. of the ventilator, which I was given to assemble at home.

Caring for Marilyn's welfare entailed making her physical life as easy and as comfortable as possible. This involved using the right equipment at the right time. Bits of kit I had ordered to make her life easier were now arriving at the door. So, over time, in came the walking sticks, wheelchair, walking frame, commode, hospital bed, hoist, wrist brace, neck brace, finger straighteners to stop her fingers from curling prematurely, foot bath, walking machine which allowed her to walk while still seated, suction machine to help her cope with uncontrollable drooling, etc. This entailed more than just making a few phone calls; they needed to be followed up. I became the shock absorber between Marilyn and those who had failed to deliver on their promises and so let her down. The usefulness of each item was short-lived, and I added each redundant item to the other useless pieces of kit in the museum of modern medical equipment I was creating.

There were other matters which also needed urgent attention. I conducted a risk assessment of the house, and called in a fire officer for advice on electrical safety and how to manoeuvre Marilyn out of the house in case of fire or other emergency. As the days passed I found it increasingly difficult to seat her on the toilet and to give her a daily shower and hair wash. New symptoms frequently appeared unannounced, demanding attention and a solution for their management.

The community matron, who had taken to referring me as Red Adair, asked how I was coping, I replied, 'I feel like a wooden stake being hammered into dry ground, and every time we are let down I feel another blow of the hammer.'

Emotional Welfare

In addition to caring for her illness and her physical needs, the problem which loomed largest in my mind was finding a way to help Marilyn ease the mental anguish she must have been undergoing. It set me thinking about how I would cope in such circumstances.

I reasoned that, should I ever become physically

incapacitated but retain my mental faculties, my way of coping with it would be to think nice thoughts and reminisce. I likened my memory bank to a Victorian apothecary whose walls were lined with little wooden drawers, each containing a different medicine.

I imagined little wooden drawers in my mind, each containing a memory from the past. When sitting idly and feeling low, I would open just one drawer and pull out from it a memory from the past. For example, I remember a boy at school who had spent his formative years in Canada playing baseball and, now that he was in England, had developed a keen interest in cricket. He was a good batsman, but with an abysmal record. Every time he hit the ball, he would drop his bat and run to the other end of the wicket; he never did get the hang of it. Too much baseball, d'ya see?

This example of an apothecary's drawers of medicine I had passed on to Marilyn some time ago, and I hope she found some solace from it. However, I knew that she had to have a trigger to lead her to open one of those boxes. She would also need (want?) stimulus from an external source which involved a 'feel good' factor, however small.

Evenings, even in the summer months, grew interminably long. Marilyn's inability to speak made the silence grow louder. I took to learning by heart songs and poems such as 'The Green Eye of the Yellow God', which I then recited to her, not only for entertainment but also as a means of directing her thoughts towards the good times of days gone by. Calypsos which would have reminded her of our holidays in the Caribbean; lyrics of songs which we had played incessantly in our student days, family Christmases, our fiftieth birthday celebrations etc.

My pattern of sleep settled to between three and a half and

four hours of sleep a night, with regular alarm calls in hourly intervals: 2.30, 3.30 and so on. Unbroken sleep became a thing of the past. At each sound of my hourly alarm clock, I would drag myself off my bed, run my head under a cold tap and, flinching at the dimmed light, steady myself, and walk gingerly down the stairs to the PEG station to administer one or more of the twenty-seven syringes of the day.

To say that I was worn to the quick would be a gross understatement. I was physically and emotionally drained. My telephone was the only meaningful access to the outside world, and to professionals who were keen to lend me their support but were prevented from doing so by COVID restrictions, though they tried their very best.

On one occasion a conversation with a member of the medical professional ended with the words, 'I wish I could do more than the little I am able to do, but I can't. I will continue to do my best. Is there anything you want?'

Fighting back the tears, I replied, 'I want my mum, she'll make it better,' and with those words ended the conversation.

I was thrashing around in the water and, having come up for air twice, I felt I was going down for the third time.

As I put the phone down, I looked at Marilyn, seated at the other end of the room, and thought of my promise to her some fifty-three years before – that I would look after her 'in sickness and in health'.

The strain of push-and-pull of compassion and care was beginning to tell. I had to get each dose right on time and without mishap and, following its application, sterilise the syringes and other equipment and prepare it in readiness for the next session. I was overstrained and worn out, and tears welled up in my eyes as I resumed the daily task of attending to her.

I distinctly remember the two occasions when I came

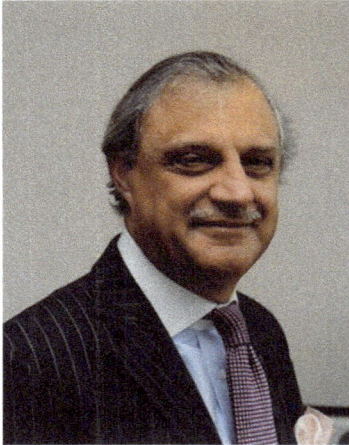

2019; before the 'Challenge'   *2021; at the tipping point*

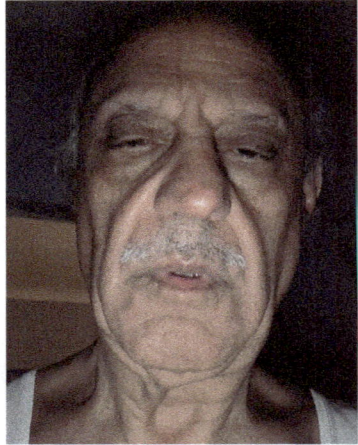

within a whisker of hitting the buffers. The awesome responsibility of being Marilyn's sole life support was taking its toll. Nevertheless, it was a solemn promise which I would keep. In any case, our love trumped the promise I had made.

True heroism … is not the urge to surpass all others at whatever cost, but the urge to serve others at whatever cost.[2]

---

[2] Arthur Ashe, quoted in *Worth Repeating* by Bob Kelly (Kregel, 2003).

Medical Support

Essentially from 2019 onwards of Marilyn's life, I was wedded to my phone. To convey how oppressive this was, I even took calls whilst on the toilet, lest I miss a 'no reply' NHS call.

The responsibility for providing much-needed physical and medical support rested with me, with support on the phone from various specialists: consultant neurologist, consultant physician for respiration and ventilation, consultant orthopaedic surgeon, GP, consultant nurse, nutritionist, speech and language therapist, neuroscience dietician specialist, community matron, clinical nurse specialist, occupational therapist, district nurse, palliative carer etc. I applied balm to her swollen joints, gave her a daily massage to soothe her aching muscles, managed equipment like the ventilator (cleaning, servicing, monitoring its use etc.), administered medication to relieve some of the symptoms, and dealt with incontinence issues, details of which I will not recount, for you would never believe me. On the first occasion Marilyn was incontinent, watching me clear up the mess, she scribbled a barely legible note to me: '*Sorry*'. I burst into tears.

The humiliation and indignity was only a part of what Marilyn suffered on a daily basis.

What follows illustrates how Marilyn suffered during those years and my struggle to overcome the trauma as I attempted to ensure that all that could be done was being done to ease her passage towards the end of her life. Given the nature of the disease, there was no knowing for how long she would have to live before her body succumbed to complete and utter physical and emotional exhaustion.

Her inability to communicate in any meaningful way led us to seemingly communicate telepathically. Psychologically, we were becoming one. Medical routine aside, I could sense what she needed when she needed it.

I was torn between being husband and carer. The distinction between wife and patient began to blur; the former was distressing and the latter stressful. There were practical difficulties. There were physical difficulties. There were emotional difficulties. I tried to do my very best for Marilyn. I prayed to God in heaven for the strength I needed to continue my efforts. Did I do enough? Could I have done more? What did I fail to do? I will never know, though there isn't a day that goes by when I don't chastise myself for, in some way, having let her down as her husband or as a carer. I tried hard, ever so hard *every day, every hour*, to strike a balance between compassion and detachment, but can't help feeling that somehow, somewhere, I must have failed her.

I have deep respect and admiration for Marilyn's resilience, deep inner strength, stoicism and the dignity with which she suffered.

The sun skipped the day on which we received the diagnosis and prognosis, and on each of the 1,185 days that followed. On the day we heard the diagnosis I felt dark clouds gathering as tears welled up inside me; they rained incessantly during those years and continue to do so intermittently to this day, and as I write this.

> *Heaven knows we need never be ashamed of our tears,*
> *for they are rain upon the blinding dust of earth,*
> *overlying our hard hearts.*[3]

---

[3] Charles Dickens, *Great Expectations*.

I watched with sadness and sorrow as the light of her life gradually turned from green to amber, and, out of sync with the other two, suddenly turned to red. The end was nigh. Until then, the degeneration had been incremental. It gradually broke Marilyn down physically, rendering her chronically, cumulatively and comprehensively imprisoned in her disabled body. Every day she died a little; every day I grieved a little.

Towards the end, the degeneration accelerated at an unprecedented pace. Attuned though I was to the unexpected, I did not expect such a rapid and serious decline within a matter of days.

In what was to be my last meaningful 'conversation' with Marilyn, I enquired:

'Are you in pain?' – she indicated 'no'.

'Are you comfortable?' – she indicated 'yes'.

'Are you afraid?' – she indicated 'no'.

In the end, when the hour finally came, I felt a tsunami of emotions that I had never allowed myself to feel. We were denied the pleasure of growing old together. One shouldn't baulk at getting old; it's a privilege denied to many. In solitary moments, such as they were, my body leaked sorrow and sadness as I constantly wondered how she must have been feeling.

Very gradually she became still. The transition from life to death seemed smooth, but there was no telling of the actual moment when she died.

On 12 June 2022, in the early hours of the morning, Marilyn, my wife of fifty-three years, answered the call of the angels.

THE AFTERMATH

Strengthen the feeble hands and make firm the feeble knees.

Isaiah 35.3

After Marilyn died I was faced with challenges of a different nature. The first order of the day was to undertake a health assessment. Given my harrowing experiences of the previous three years, it was more than likely that my health would have suffered, possibly irreparably.

With the help of my GP, I underwent a full health check, ECG, blood tests etc. On reviewing the results, my GP nodded and muttered, 'This doesn't seem to be right; everything seems to be normal. Just to make sure, I will refer you to a cardiologist because the equipment they have at the Epsom General is more sophisticated than the one we have here at the surgery. I am keen to see if your heart is sound.'

The cardiologist plugged me into a large machine which made strange sounds and spat out bits of paper. She looked at the graphs, nodded and, after reading the letter of referral again, looked at me and said, 'Everything seems to be fine.' So saying, she reached into a drawer in her desk and pulled out something which most of us haven't seen for a very long time: an old-fashioned stethoscope!

And so began the old routine: shirt off, stethoscope on my chest, 'breathe in, breathe out,' stethoscope on my back, 'breathe in, breathe out' etc. She unplugged the stethoscope from her ears and said, 'I detect a slight murmur.' After she had explained what that meant, I replied that it seemed quite natural, given that my heart was seventy-five years old. Nevertheless, she suggested that it was something that needed to be monitored.

I was pleased but felt that, given what I had been through, I was likely to have been scarred. What the scars were, and how deep they ran, time would tell.

The 'scar' has since revealed itself in the physical form of a tear in the membrane of my right eye, which can be caused by heavy lifting: in this case lifting Marilyn. At the onset of MND, Marilyn was advised to eat as much food high in protein as possible to increase her weight. So I cooked everything with cream, cheese, butter, eggs etc., and as a consequence she ballooned from her regular weight of approximately 76 kg to an eyewatering 84 kg. I'm told that lifting a 'dead weight' is equivalent to lifting twice the actual weight.

If left untreated, a tear such as the one in my eye can lead to a detached retina, which in turn can cause loss of sight. Should it come to that, and if surgery can't fix it, then so be it; it is a price worth paying.

Physical wellbeing having been dealt with, I now turned my attention to my emotional state. I found the silence in the house foreboding, and began suffering from an adverse reaction to an empty chair amongst occupied chairs in familiar surroundings. The unoccupied passenger seat in the car, the unoccupied chair at the breakfast and dinner table, the unoccupied chair in front of the television, an unoccupied chair in front of the live fire in the sitting room, an unoccupied chair at a function I had recently attended. This was not because of my missing the person I loved; it was because the empty chair was bereft of a friend, a companion, a relative – in short, of an individual. It symbolised how lonesome (which is not the same as being lonely) one can be, even when surrounded by people.

It very quickly became clear that I should go out as much as possible and meet as many people as possible. With this in mind, I joined various groups, including a walking group for those who were recently bereaved. The walks tended to be where one was surrounded by lots of green and blue: trees, grass, lakes, rivers etc. They were fairly well attended, usually by between eight and twelve people. On the few walks I attended, save for one exception, I was the only male and the youngest there. Most of the women present were in their eighties. The walks were a very good idea because one could talk freely; we were all in it together.

What I learned during those walks was that, as a general rule, women are more resilient and more able to cope with bereavement than men. By and large, the generation of women of which I speak were full-time housewives in the traditional sense; they did not go out to work to earn a living, and so, upon the death of their spouses, the pattern of their daily life didn't change much. In the normal course of events, they would wake up in the morning, make breakfast for their husband and see him off to work. The rest of the day until his return would be taken up with their daily routine: working for a charity, shopping, cleaning, cooking, washing up, doing the laundry, general housework. In the evening, they would cook supper, watch television with their spouse and retire for the night. The pattern would repeat itself the following day and so on.

They were self-sufficient, and in that sense they were ahead of the curve.

Furthermore, for many widowhood brought a bonus; they could have a lie-in of a morning, there was no further need to cook breakfast and supper at set times, the TV remote was now firmly in their grasp, and they controlled the thermostat; no longer did they have to hear their spouses say, 'Oh, do stop complaining about the cold, Julia; just throw another rope of pearls around your neck!' The widowers, on the other hand, tend to flounder. They can't cook, operate the washing machine etc., and 'man flu' quickly becomes a thing of the past. I'm not that saying it is all beer and skittles for widows, but for them the daily grind does seem less of a grind.

I tired of the walks soon enough. The final straw came when, turning up one morning for a walk, I was approached by a member of the group with a leaflet and the words, 'Do you have trouble with strength and balance?' To my undying shame, I replied 'Only after I've had a wee dram.' This did not endear me to her. Although they continued to invite me, this last exchange was an indication that I was ready to move on.

To help me recover, I made arrangements for the house, which had suffered five years of neglect, to be redecorated to give it a lift, and to eliminate the damage to paintwork, plasterwork and woodwork, of which I was the principal cause as I wheeled Marilyn and various equipment around. Although this damage was not noticeable to visitors, I was acutely aware of it, and it served as a constant reminder of the past.

Many suggested that I get a dog: something which I found incomprehensible. I was in no mood, on coming home, to be met by a dog's cry of 'woof, woof', i.e. 'where is my dinner and take me for a walk'; I was desperate to be greeted by a warm, welcoming voice asking me how my day had gone and with whom I could have an ordinary conversation. I thought about getting a parrot, but my childhood experience of an African Grey reminded me that they have a gift of picking up passing conversation and a habit of swearing. In any event, pets require attention, they are high-maintenance, and I was at a stage where it was *I* who required attention, it was *I* who was 'high-maintenance' and it was *I* who wanted to be welcomed. I dreaded the absence of another heartbeat in the house — of no one to bless me whenever I sneezed.

The daily grind and household chores were beginning to have an adverse effect on me. The thought of sitting down on a Sunday morning to write a week's menu of twenty-one meals was daunting. Marilyn and I were in the habit of planning the forthcoming week's menu of three squares a day each Sunday morning after breakfast. I couldn't face it on my own and realised that I would slide into the habit of living off ready-to-cook meals, which are far from nutritional if consumed on a daily basis.

In a fit of introspection, I sat down with pencil and paper and, treating myself as a patient, asked myself aloud, 'What is your problem?'

I drew two columns. In one I made a list of those things which I found to be a chore and wanted to avoid. Whist I had done those things for Marilyn willingly, I resented having to do them for myself. In the other column I listed those things which I had previously enjoyed doing, and which would afford me a good chance of recovery. And guess what? Off the page a possible solution: engage someone who would do more around the house than merely clean. This, surely, would deal with most of the issues in the first column which were troubling me, and leave me to concentrate on starting to live life again. We all have two lives; the second life begins when we realise that we have only one life.

I began to look into engaging a housekeeper. With the problems of Brexit and COVID, there was a dearth of cleaners and, although there was a small army of unemployed, they were not necessarily employable. The thought of interviewing, training and selecting someone was daunting, and the possibility that they might prove to be unsuitable and consequently the whole process would have to start again was putting me off. I couldn't face the disruption it necessitated. Being fastidious by nature, I knew it was going to be a hard post to fill.

To make the vetting process easier, I visited four hotels and enquired of their housekeepers whether any of their staff had a few hours a week to spare for me. I was met with the response that they themselves were so short-staffed that their staff were being asked to work double shifts.

I asked any cleaners I came across if they had spare capacity or knew colleagues or friends who might be interested, only to be met with a negative response. The answer was the same if I spoke to the householders rather than the cleaners themselves. An uncharitable thought occurred to me: were my friends being disingenuous and protecting their vested interest? 'Cleaners are like gold dust,' I kept being told on enquiry. I remember my father advising me, 'On no account should you disclose the identity of your tailor, accountant or bookmaker.' In the twenty-first century, this seems to apply to cleaners as well.

I looked in the classified columns of various local papers and visited the local paper shop to see if anybody was advertising for work, but this met with little success. Indeed, it is now rare to find a newspaper shop which displays postcards in its window advertising one's requirements.

A friend suggested that I should advertise. This was an alien concept to me, and I vacillated, partly because I really did not know where to begin. What sort of advertising, and in what media? The parish magazine, the local paper, going online? The last was out of the question. I based my excuse for doing nothing on the grounds that, as it was a 'seller's market', anyone who was halfway decent would already be gainfully employed.

A friend phoned to say that she had seen some postcards advertising for cleaners in the window of a sub-post office in the next town, and that I should go there and place in their window a card advertising my need for a cleaner. 'What have you got to lose?' she asked in exasperation.

Having now run out of excuses, and as a matter of courtesy to her, I took myself off to the shop, and … lo and behold, there were no fewer than seven advertisements looking for a cleaner. I felt I had to give it a go but was at a loss for what to write. In the end I decided to cast the net as wide as possible and started drafting an advertisement on a postcard.

Just as I was about to finish, I hit a brick wall; I froze. I didn't want to advertise my mobile number, but, of course, I knew that I had no option. However, I drew the line at advertising my name as well. After much ruminating, a cunning plan emerged as to how I could disassociate my name from my phone number. The solution was for me to give a false name, and even more cunning was the name I chose – *Lesley* –

thinking that, as a unisex name it wouldn't frighten the horses. I didn't have the nous to realise that the way the name is spelt is an indicator of the gender. Oh, well, one can't get everything right.

The newsagent's rate for an advertisement on a postcard was 92p a week. (Why in heaven's name 92p? Whyever not £1? But that's a story for another day.) I took a deep breath, struggled to release my postcard into the grasping hand of the newsagent and, in a rush of blood to the head, decided to go the whole hog and bought a month's advertising! Spendthrift that I am, I handed over the princely sum of £3.68 in coin of the realm – untraceable, d'you see?

> *WANTED*
> *Cleaner/housekeeper*
>
> *Days: Negotiable*
> *Hours: Negotiable*
> *Live in/live out*
> *Part time/full time*
> *Pay: Negotiable (above minimum wage)*
> *Start date: Negotiable*
>
> *Interested?*
> *Call or text: 123 456 78901*
>
> *Lesley*

As you can see, dear reader, the net could not have been cast wider. I still say it was the best advert on show; it stood head and shoulders above the others – because it was mine!

A simple enough story, but its importance is to convey that however trifling the issue may seem, it loomed large, was serious to me and taxed my mental resources.

Needless to say I heard nothing, until then one day as I was at the hob, stirring my gruel for lunch, the phone rang and a voice at the other end said, 'Can I speak to Lesley?'

Not recognising the name, I answered curtly that I knew no one by that name and promptly hung up, muttering to myself, 'Well, bless my soul, wretched double-glazing salesmen calling at mealtimes.' (Well, words in Anglo-Saxon to that effect.)

As luck would have it, a couple of minutes later I received a text message: *Lesley, I phoned you just now but you put the phone down. I'm sure I have the right number as this is the number you advertised for a cleaner.* The penny dropped; I twigged what it was all about, had a meaningful conversation with her and, following an interview, engaged Olena Kozyra, whose importance becomes clear later.

The next step in my rehabilitation was to get out and meet as many people as possible, so I joined various groups. Marilyn and I used to play canasta regularly every week. I enquired about joining a group who played cards locally. I discovered that they played on a Monday morning between ten o'clock and noon – at which I thought, *Who plays cards at ten o'clock on a Monday morning? That's when I'm coming home after a night out.* That was the end of that.

I joined a number of other groups but met with little success. The problem wasn't that they were being difficult. There was nothing wrong with the individuals concerned, all of whom were without exception very welcoming; the problem lay with *me*. I had to grasp the nettle and face my demons instead of kicking the can down the road.

I had previously seen the future as a friend; now I saw it as a stranger. I felt my future leaving me behind.

It seems to be a universally acknowledged fact that friends and relations who rally round after bereavement tend to fade away after six months, get on with their lives and assume that you are doing the same. The consequences of this are predicated on the circumstances surrounding the death of a loved one and the character of the bereaved. Having said that, all my friends were kind, caring, considerate and nonjudgemental.

Invitations dried up as friends got on with their usual round of social engagements. There is something about the chattering classes that abhors odd numbers. They are loath to invite anyone who does not form a couple. Marilyn and I were never troubled by odd numbers. In fact, it was usually the 'odd' bod or boddess who made the evening more interesting. I made greater effort and did a good deal more entertaining than I had previously, but this only worked as long as my guests reciprocated within a reasonable timeframe. In some cases it was months before they were in touch again; it left great gaps in my diary.

Fourteen hours are a great many hours to fill every day. Forward planning became a necessity. Being alone meant I needed to work very hard, which I did. It was time-consuming, it was expensive and it was tiring. In the end I gave up making the running. I no longer had the energy, the enthusiasm or the inclination to be the one who would always make the effort of organising social get-togethers.

My desire to make new friends and cultivate acquaintances was born out of a belief that it would easier to converse with new friends naturally. They would be unaware of my backstory and so, unlike existing friends, wouldn't feel they were treading on eggshells when talking to me. I resolved to move forward to the sound of a trumpet, not that of a soulful tune played on the smallest violin.

My attempts at cultivating existing friendships and making new friends met with limited success, given that friends, for whatever reason, did not introduce me to their friends. Marilyn and I had always gone to great lengths to introduce our friends to others. It wasn't helping me to widen my circle of friends, which would have enabled me to spend time amongst like-minded people, something that the walks didn't do. It was clear that I was on my own when it came to expanding my social circle.

Under normal circumstances, the matter of 'new' friends would not have been an issue, but in this case, with isolation during the pandemic and having been out of circulation for three years, the social landscape had changed. So I persevered at becoming socially active. During a period of two months I hosted or organised no fewer than thirty-seven social engagements.

I was lonesome, not lonely. The deadly silence of which I have written was closing in on me. Although I seemed good-humoured, at the back of each smile there was a tear all the while and a heartache that no one could see. There was a ring on my finger, but my heart ached inside. I needed to move on from dwelling on the nightmare of the past and start thinking of the future, but the past kept intruding and my mind wandered towards speculating on the nature of my inevitable death.

The medical profession, with the best of intentions, is busy concentrating on 'improving the quality of life' of the elderly, and so sets about fixing things that go wrong often as a natural consequence of old age. Knee replacements, pacemakers, hearing aids, hip replacements, bypasses, medication (for cholesterol, diabetes etc.), a cocktail of vitamin infusions and stem cell therapy. We take 'preventative' measures – cancer screening, DNA testing, urine analysis, blood tests – all in an effort to chase the elixir of youth. Small wonder, then, that so many of us are carried away by something nasty such as Alzheimer's, cancer or Parkinson's ... and now the demon of motor neuron disease has reared its ugly head. Extremely rare though it is at the time of writing, It won't be long before it too becomes commonplace. I have seen its ugly horns close up; it is no respecter of age, and it imprisons its victims.

Are we all becoming coffin dodgers?

I remember clearly the eve of the millennium when, as the clock approached midnight, my host at a dinner party turned on the radio to welcome in the new year. The proverbial pips of midnight were followed by the news. The newscaster announced that the first millennium baby in the UK had been born at two minutes past midnight and that scientists believed she had every possibility of living to be 200 years old. After a brief silence, the conversation around the dinner table went thus:

'That's astonishing!'

'I don't see why. People are already living to the age of ninety, so it is quite possible that in a hundred years' time they will live to be 200.'

'I wouldn't want to live for 200 years. Who would want to live to be 200?'

'Everyone who is 199!'

... and therein lies the conundrum.

Being in the presence of other people in a work environment would have helped a great deal, but I had resigned from my legal consultancy and non-executive directorships at the outset and, although my former non-executive directorships had been restored after Marilyn died, the role was far from challenging or time-consuming. I applied to three charities to work on a volunteer basis, offering to do whatever they had on offer, sweeping floors, washing dishes, making tea etc., but the work offers never materialised. Former lawyers wandering about the place, whatever their task, had little appeal. In reality I lacked the necessary skills, or perhaps I was just too honest at interviews.

The story goes that an interview for a job was going very well. To round off the interview, the interviewer asked the candidate, 'What would say is your greatest weakness?'

'My greatest weakness is that I am dead honest.'

'I don't think that's a weakness.'

'I don't give a monkey's what you think.'

Abrupt end of interview.

Indulging in leisure activities such as reading, listening to music or watching television resulted in my mind wandering off and dwelling on the past. As I am gregarious by nature, such solo activities were of limited value.

I decided to visit friends in Yorkshire for a few days. I set out fearing an empty passenger seat on a long journey. The problem with motorway driving is that it is boring and leads one to dwell on things. How I miss those not infrequent lively 'exchanges' with Marilyn in the car when we were at odds about which turning I should have taken! If, dear reader, you are no stranger to this phenomenon, I implore you to cherish it. It won't last forever; it's later than you think.

Music didn't help, as some of it evoked strong memories of the past. Although the visit was successful, the drive was not. It made me realise that I was not yet ready to invoke my much-cherished plans for visiting various friends around the country.

Given the paucity of new introductions, I was now left to fend for myself. I decided to take a 'proper' holiday abroad, where I could be in the midst of others; a change of atmosphere would do me good. After all, what did I have to lose?

And that, dear reader, leads you to the diary entries I kept during my trip on the Rhine.

COPING WITH GRIEF AND EXORCISING DEMONS

When sorrows come, they come not as single spies but in battalions.

Shakespeare, *Hamlet*

Not wanting to fly, or to holiday in an environment populated by wives, sweethearts[4] canoodling in a corner and happy families, I settle for a cruise on the River Rhine departing from Cologne. On this occasion, the cruise is designed for those who want to travel on their own: 'singletons' in modern parlance. There is only one passenger per cabin and, unlike normal cruising, no single supplement is charged for the trip. I pat myself on the back for having this Klieg moment.

I travel to Paris on Eurostar. We must be the only nation in the world which spends squillions on establishing an international train station but does not provide drop-off and pick-up facilities for its passengers.

I am not after a 'Club Med' experience, nor the equivalent of a summer rave on Mykonos:[5] just a few days on water in

---

[4] 'Wives and sweethearts – may they never meet': Saturday toast in the Royal Navy wardroom.

[5] This should not be taken as indicative of a misspent youth.

the company of undemanding like-minded people on holiday, to reset my compass. Thereafter I plan to settle down to enjoy the bare essentials of a civilised existence: a roof over one's head, the constituent ingredients of an expertly constructed dry martini, and some Thedgeley's chunky-cut 'Olde Tyme' marmalade, a pot of coffee and burnt toast. I am looking to develop a lifestyle which enhances my presence as I enter the 'metallic years': silver in my hair, gold in my teeth, and lead in my bottom.

... and so it comes to pass that I embark on the MV *Weeping Willows* on what, in many ways, turns out to be a unique trip on a river in a land where they count distance in kilometres.

What happens on the boat[6] grievously undermines the purpose of my having taken the trip. The bitter experience is firmly etched in my mind. It is blindingly obvious that what happened could have been foreseen by anyone with foresight.[7]

If you get the impression that I'm being economic with the actualité, you'd be right. I'm also aware that in so doing I am slipping into Instagram mode and concealing a more sombre reality.

In the words of Nicholas-Sebastian Chamort: 'Of all days, the one most surely wasted is the one on which one has not laughed.'[8] The bouts of humour depicted here mask the acute distress and upset I experienced on this trip. Suffice it to say that the holiday has stress-tested my sense of humour to its limits.

---

[6] A note for landlubbers: a vessel which sails on a river is called a boat (as is a submarine), not a ship.

[7] A statement which is blindingly obvious itself.

[8] *Maximes et penséés*, 1796.

Those of you who are landlubbers may appreciate my subtle introduction of nautical terms in the vain hope that this will prove to be a mind-improving book.

For reasons which will become apparent, I kept a journal on the trip, and what follows is a reworked and expanded version of it. It is written in the present tense to lend it a sense of immediacy.

The written style of this chapter is different from what you have read earlier, because I have reproduced the narrative here as it appears in my journal. The earlier chapters were written more than a year after I had written the diary and should have really been rewritten for the sake of consistency, but I just can't be fussed with rewriting them. Little seems to have changed since my school days, which were best summed up by one of my housemaster's mid-term reports: *Ishani and his nose have yet to meet the grindstone this term.*

As you see, a predisposition to cut corners has not deserted me. So my advice to those amongst you who are of a literary bent, is to grit your teeth and bear it, and to those of you who are pedants, get over it.

You will find the diary an easy read; you will have read these words before, but not in the order in which they appear here.

Day 1

On the day of my departure, as I'm in the process of packing for the trip, I receive a phone call from my therapist, who wants to be reassured that all is well and that I haven't got cold feet (such mutterings have been voiced). I assure her that I am in the process of packing as we speak and promise to give her a full debriefing on my return. She enquires about the dress code. 'Smart casual,' I reply, adding, 'However, I'm packing my silk dressing gown; I feel lucky!' I have already had the velvet on my slippers crushed the week before.

The first problem of the day: it's been five years since I went on holiday, and so I forget that Eurostar now leaves not from Waterloo but from St Pancras, a mere million miles from the ole' homestead, thereby increasing my travel time by a good hour and a half. What's worse, Eurostar requires passengers to check in two hours before departure – *two* hours! For pity's sake, it's a train! We now live in a world where trains think they are planes, private clubs boast restaurants instead of dining rooms and restaurants pretend to be clubs (viz. the Coriander Club, an Indian restaurant in Hampstead).

Having been warned about the dire quality of the fare on offer on board, I venture into a 'steak bar' and 'wait to be seated'. I eventually catch the eye of a spotty yoof (he must be all of thirty-five years old) masquerading as a waiter, lounging at the back of the room in a mouldy T-shirt, idly excavating his nose with the tip of his index finger. I order a steak and salad. He asks if I want wine.

'Yes, please,' I reply.

'Red or white, sir?'

'A glass of red, please.'

'In that case, I recommend a sauvignon blanc.'

I sigh. He comes back with my steak and I enquire, 'Why is your thumb on my steak?'

'To stop it falling on the floor again, sir,' comes the reply.

Let's blame Brexit for the acute shortage of skilled labour.

I still have an hour to kill and so look for somewhere to sit. The few seats available in the departure hall are all occupied, save for three chairs in a cordoned-off seating area displaying pictorial signs of:

- a pregnant woman,
- an old man walking with the aid of a stick, and
- an individual in a wheelchair.

Really? Why would anyone who is already in a chair have need of another?

Once more, I am struck by a lightbulb moment. I immediately develop a stoop and a limp and help myself to a seat. Yet again, I pat myself on the back and finger my debit card in readiness to pay a fine to a member of the railway Stasi should it become necessary. I didn't get where I am today by not being in business for myself.

I clamber aboard and take my allocated seat opposite an elderly woman who is wearing a face covering – possibly as a habit from the days of the pandemic. As I look at her I am puzzled. I have never previously had to concentrate so hard on a person's face, but on this occasion I look hard for some clue as to what her face looks like, because only her eyes are visible. I wonder, do dull eyes betray what lies underneath the covering? In this case, does the face match her lovely eyes? How on earth do Arabs manage? Is beauty overrated?

Of course, there are many people who are attractive without being beautiful, just as there are beauties who bore, and the danger of beauty in the very young is that it can make the business of life seem deceptively easy for them.

Of the four great gifts that the fairies may or may not bring to the christening – Brains, Birth, Beauty and Money – it is Beauty that makes closed doors spring open at a touch, whether it is for a job interview, a place at a dining table, a brilliant promotion or a lift home. Everyone, regardless of their gender or their sexual proclivity, would always rather deal with a good-looking face than one which is not.

And no one is more aware of this than the beauties themselves. They have a power they simultaneously respect and take for granted. Despite the moralists who tut-tut about its transience, it is generally a power that is never completely lost.

… and what when old age sets in? Prettiness fades and seldom leaves a trace of its former self. However, in the case of someone who was a beauty in her youth, one can usually trace in the wrinkled lines of a nonagenarian, stooped and leaning on a stick, the style and confidence that turned heads in a ballroom in 1929.

The lunch trolley trundles to a stop near the masked woman and she partakes of a pastry. To eat this she lowers her face mask to reveal a beauty which matches her grey-blue eyes. She is charming and erudite. I learn of what great pleasure can be derived from beauty when it is *revealed*.

The journey progresses smoothly, and I arrive at the Gare

du Nord in one piece and in relative peace. I disembark and follow the river boat company's instructions to foregather under their flag at the entrance to the platform. Feeling somewhat embarrassed, I station myself some small distance from the flag in a vain attempt to disassociate myself from the ever-growing polyester crowd gathering under it, encased in plastic quilted coats, wearing gym shoes ('trainers', they call them) like latter-day Teddy Boys. Whatever happened to Dunn & Co, Crombie, Harris Tweed, Austin Reed and the duffel coat? I look generally in the opposite direction, nonchalantly humming a nondescript tune to give the impression that I am idly waiting for someone.

The tour manager (I wince, for I have booked independently through my travel agent, who made no mention of any 'tour') points towards the exit. As luck would have it, it is close to where I am standing, and so I am at the head of the queue wending its way towards the coach which has been summoned to transport us to the boat moored at Cologne.

It is raining, but I stand back in the rain, to the bemusement of the other passengers, whose suitcases are being loaded as they clamber aboard. There is method in my madness, dear reader, for when we come to disembark my suitcase is the first to be unloaded and I am collecting the key to my stateroom whilst the others wait in the rain for their suitcases. The fecundity of my mind terrifies me.

The journey across Paris is interesting. Riots are in full swing. The Parisians are complaining about police brutality;[9]

---

[9] Earlier in the week, *Le Monde* had carried a photo and narrative of a policeman shooting dead a shoplifter emerging from a supermarket.

the usual mayhem ensues with vehicles overturned, tyres burning, bonfires alight in the middle of roads etc. We are assured that Hussein, our coach driver, knows his way around Paris and will avoid the rioting even if it means driving around the Périphérique!

As we approach a road junction, Hussein asks us to look to the right if we want to catch a glimpse of the riot, and of police breaking heads as they weigh into the rioters. Inspector Clouseau it is not.

The passenger sitting beside me seems to be possessed of the antiseptic self-assurance of an OFSTED inspector. She shakes her head and asks why it is that the French are such an irascible and emotional race, prone to violence at the slightest provocation. I explain that I attribute this not to psychological factors but rather to physiological ones; it's because they don't eat Marmite, I say.[10]

'And they don't drink tea,' she adds.

'That would explain why their per capita productivity is seven percent higher than that of UK "workers", I reply with mild sarcasm.

She mumbles her name, 'Tara ...' but I don't catch what follows. The short exchange leaves me guessing her surname. I chuckle and bestow on her a double-barrelled one: Raboom-Diyaeh.

She hails from Ecclesfield, home of the famous 'cakes'. She is here on the recommendation of her therapist to help her overcome her aquaphobia.

---

[10] Marmite contains B vitamins (amongst other things), which increase levels of a brain-calming neurotransmitter.

After a brief moment's silence, she asks, 'Boats sink, don't they?'

I reply, and in a fit of poor judgement, hoping to settle her nerves, I continue, 'Yes, but only once'.

Silence ensues as she contemplates the deep meaning of my reply, while I settle down with my copy of *Chekhov's Short Stories*. She glances at the title and says, 'I didn't know you were a Trekkie.' It takes a moment for the penny to drop. I feel like someone who is holding a first-class ticket and suddenly finds himself sitting next to a lunatic.

I take a close look at her and wonder about the history of her frock. It's obviously an old favourite. She was wise to remove the curtain rings – lovely fabric; she was lucky to find so much of it. Well, so much for erudite conversation. I'm filled with a sense of foreboding.

On arrival, I am escorted to my cabin and begin unpacking, feeling mightily pleased with myself. The silk dressing gown is the first garment to cosset a waiting hanger. I hum 'Good Vibrations'[11] whilst unpacking.

The *Weeping Willows* carries only seventy-one passengers. It looks promising that we'll make a party of it. However, it's not long before I realise that I am one of the youngest on board and that the average age is in excess of seventy-eight years. Of the seventy-one fellow travellers there are only five men, including me; the rest appear to be dour, glum-looking women, most of whom are loners, avowed spinsters, divorcees or widows (some recent). With some possible exceptions, they are not as young as they are painted.

---

[11] Apologies to the Rolling Stones.

- Some have woken up to the fact that life has passed them by and are bitter.

- Some are commitment-phobes.

- Some are narcissists hankering after the willpower to pursue dating apps.

- Some are struggling with decoding life's social norms.

- Some have simply let themselves go and given up.

There is an announcement that there is no doctor or pharmacy on board, because the boat moors every day at a town where a doctor and pharmacy are generally readily accessible. The announcer's voice, tightly wound, comes out at the speed of the terms and conditions at the end of a radio advertisement.

Passengers are also informed that the small button with a red light, to be found in each cabin and generally dotted around the boat, is *not* for summoning room service (there is none); it is an emergency call button. Hmmm.

Conversation noise levels are high, as many passengers are hard of hearing. They wander about cupping their ears in a ball of concentration in an effort to improve the pitch and timbre of the speech they are receiving. The most common phrase to be heard is 'whaddya say?'

This is going to be a challenge sans pareil.

The length of the dining saloon is something to behold. The buffet table at the centre is so long that it disappears with the curvature of the Earth.

This evening, dinner consists of a dish I don't recognise. I am dazzled by the intense dark green wonder of the dish, which reminds me of a parsley and tomato soup I once had at a youth hostel during my student days in deepest Scotland. Perhaps I am too much in a temps perdu, but it summons another old memory of a Kentish boy's dish involving bread, layers of crisps, tinned tuna and condensed milk.

At dinner a fellow passenger informs me that she is here on respite and that her husband is terminally ill. I offer my sympathy and, being the dolt that I am, I enquire after his condition.

This elicits a blow-by-blow description of the various stages of his illness and how stressful it all is: trying to manoeuvre him off his bed onto his wheelchair, dealing with his incontinence, giving him his daily wash, lifting him up after a fall etc. Apparently, throughout his life he had divided his time between watching the racing channel, half a bottle of whiskey and sixty Benson & Hedges, resulting in a lung disease that brought forth the most spectacular explosive fits of coughing.

I know all about caring for someone who is terminally ill and don't need to be reminded of it. I feel myself approaching a precipice and try to dismiss haunting images.

Being a neophyte at this sort of thing, I try to calm her by resting my hand on her arm in what I consider to be a perfectly safe, non-threatening, well-meaning gesture. Fortunately, she doesn't raise the alarm for attempted assault, and the fear of having my collar felt dissipates.

The encounter at dinner leaves me shaken. It brings back memories of the occasion when Marilyn was at the washbasin, holding on to it to steady herself. In the nanosecond it took me to reach for a tissue, the muscles in her legs collapsed without any warning and she fell to the floor, striking her head on the rim of the basin on her way down. She lay there on the bathroom floor bleeding profusely from the head wound.

There were no paramedics available for at least two hours. I was advised to stem the flow of blood as quickly as possible before taking her to A&E. Given that during COVID a visit to A&E was not an option, a nurse on the phone talked me through the process of applying pressure to the wound to stem the flow of blood, cleaning it and stitching the wound as best I could by using a technique employed by surgeons (and on the battlefield) as an alternative to dissolvable stitches.

Raising my emotional shield as high as I could, I looked up to the heavens and prayed that the stitches would hold. By now my hands were shaking; I was soaked in sweat and fearful of not knowing if what I was doing was right. Mercifully, it was, but it's not an experience I want to repeat. This was not a case of 'if you've done it once, you can do it again' ... or was it?

> *I am only one, but I am one. I cannot do everything, but I can do something. And because I cannot do everything, I will not refuse to do the something that I can do.*[12]

I head at warp speed straight for the bar and a large Glenlivet. I ask for two doubles – both in the same glass – and weep into it.

... and so to bed, in trepidation of what lies in store over the next seven days.

---

[12] Edward Everett Hale.

Day 2

Not a good start to the day, as I discover that temporary amnesia can reliably be induced by placing one's head immediately beneath an open drawer.

Notwithstanding yesterday's sad encounter with a fellow passenger, I resolve to be positive, cheerful and optimistic.

The waiters, who all hail from the Baltic, are well-groomed courteous and speak perfect English: a welcome change from the natives of the UK. The captain, who is French, refers to the UK as 'Brexit Island'. We engage in some light banter. She asks about the relationship between England and Scotland, which she can't fathom. I explain that it is a union by consent of both kingdoms. She then mentions Ireland. Anxious not to get involved in a conversation on geopolitics, I explain in simple terms that the United Kingdom comprises four nations: Scotland, whose people like to keep everything they have and anything else they can lay their hands on; Wales, whose people prey on their knees and on their neighbours; Northern Ireland, whose people have no principles but are willing to die for them, and England, a nation of self-made people, which is a blessing because it absolves God from all blame.

The dining service, while not servile, is friendly, and the food high-flown but not flashily presented. This being Germany, there are no 'New World' wines on the list, but some good German ones. However, none of the classics. Whatever happened to those classics from Germany (Blue Nun, Black Tower) and Portugal (Mateus Rosé)?

The passengers continue not to impress and refuse steadfastly to decompress.[13] The weather is turning decidedly cool and wet.

---

[13] A nautical term. The reader can expect many more to come.

I'm nonplussed at being approached by women to whom I have not been formally introduced, wanting to engage me in conversation. Formal introductions, I gather, are a thing of the past; one simply rocks up and says, 'Hi.' I'm reminded of the stricture of my therapist for having been born in the wrong century; it's a cross I bear with what little dignity I can muster.

Conversation with my fellow inmates is becoming increasingly difficult, as none of them are like-minded. There is much talk about their children, grandchildren, cats, dogs and gibbons, not necessarily in that order. They are all, without exception, possessed of a high propensity to whip out pictures of their grandchildren from their purses faster than Wyatt Earp's draw at the OK Corral.

Of the other four male passengers, two are members of an angling club and stick together, regaling each other with war stories about their angling experience. The third, who rejoices in the double-barrelled name of Howard Watford-Bypass, is a recently divorced gentleman of the old school. Prone to shooting his cuffs, he is immaculately dressed and well-groomed. I discern a faint whiff of hair pomade. He had been married for many a year. He is whiter than I've ever seen before: a man of pale complexion, even, I suspect, when (if ever) he is full of the joys of life. He looks like a blood donor who couldn't say no. If his pyjamas are not double-breasted and embroidered with the family cypher, I'm a parsnip.

From his barrel tummy to his curlicued accent, Howard is a collector's item. A man of dour disposition who'd knock the joie out of your vivre as soon as look at you, and yet … and yet I can't help thinking, *Here's a gander who'll meander in search of a goose.*

I ask him what keeps him busy.

'Oh, this and that. Import, export, you know the sort of thing.'

'Indeed I do,' I mutter under my breath. Fortunes are made but never quite banked. As slippery as the stone of a ripe avocado. He gives me the impression of one who is always at the airport when his ship comes in. A man who is as honest as the day is long on the twenty-first day of December.

He ponders why what he thought was a marriage made in heaven had unravelled in the manner it did. Although they had been stepping out for some time, he was not convinced that she was a kindred spirit until she casually remarked over lunch one day that she thought Shane Warne was 'giving the ball more flight these days'. It was at that moment that he was moved to propose to his girlfriend, he said.

He considers the matter for a while and advances his theory as to why so many marriages fail. With an episcopal pause, waiting for his sermon to echo off the furthest apse of some imagined cathedral, he adds that he feels the knell sounding on his monastic life and that it may be time to move towards les plaisirs d'amour. *Hmm*, I think, *perhaps a gander after all*. Anyway, who am I to judge.

Incidentally, you may be interested to learn that the first testicular guard used in cricket was in 1874, and the first helmet was used one hundred years later in 1974. It took a hundred years for cricketers to realise that the brain is also important ... but clearly not as important as their 'crown jewels'. Makes one wonder.

Dinner kicks off with French onion soup.

A fellow diner sits down beside me and introduces herself

as Heanor Hucknall; the name sounds familiar, but I can't place it. She asks the steward, 'What is this? It's not that soup which has toast floating on it, is it? I don't drink soup with bread and cheese in it.'

She's served French onion soup sans pain grillé. She then pronounces the soup to be too hot and so adds water to it from her drinking glass to cool it.

I resist the temptation to bury my head in my hands. I'm in for a long haul.

For someone who is itching to leave the table as soon as he can, the next course takes far too long to arrive. That's fine if you're sitting on a boat off Sardinia, tucking into a plate of olives, on your third bottle of prosecco of the morning, and watching topless hookers diving off Silvio Berlusconi's yacht and swimming madly for shore with their passports between their teeth.

The pork with cockles in white wine sauce which follows the soup is a little disconcerting. No wonder Leviticus declares a double prohibition.

Dessert for Heanor involves grabbing a handful of grapes from a bowl of fruit and drooling over them like an aged maiden aunt trying to find a walnut whip in a box of chocolates. These she proceeds to peel, as carefully as one peels a sticking plaster off an open wound, and pops into her mouth one at a time. She exudes a gracelessness born of egalitarianism.

What I need is a change of scene. I go up on deck for some fresh air in an attempt to stem the emotion welling up in me, brought about by the simple motion of her peeling grapes.

I stand there on my own, wrapped up against the cold wind, damp from earlier rainfall, staring at the sky devoid of moon and stars. I miss the cry of seagulls, the heat of the day and the glow of the moon, which I had foolishly eagerly anticipated when this boat set sail. The clear waters I see are made opaque by the pollution of recent memories. The moon and stars no longer shine.

Heanor and her grapes trigger the recollection of a moment when Marilyn had lost her ability to swallow. All food and water was taken in liquid form through tubes into her stomach. This, combined with the effect of medication to stop the uncontrollable saliva which constantly cascaded from her mouth, left her tongue parched and bereft of all taste. To ease Marilyn's discomfort, I would peel a grape, insert a Q-tip through one end and ever so gently rub the grape back and forth on her tongue to moisten it, to give her some little relief from the dryness and also give her a sense of taste. Time and again I would mutter to myself, 'She deserves better than this.'

Acutely distressing though it was, I persevered with the grapes and in so doing sought to bring her some comfort in some small degree. Dark days indeed.

I find myself singing in a low whisper, just as I used to sing to her.

You should have liveried vassals
Attending to you night and day
Waving fans with their hands
Just to brush your blues away.

You should have someone who loves you
Standing by to peel your grapes
And who'll remain
To do whatever it takes.

If I had the riches of Arabia
I would give you all I own, but I can tell you
That I love you,
Love you to the nth degree.

And if you have
What you should have
It'll never come close
To the love I have for you.

Despite my well-intentioned resolution of earlier this morning, try as I might, I struggle to look on the bright side.

I head to the bar for an absinthe. I retire for the night three sheets to the wind.

Day 3

Pray, why is it that people think I'm a doctor? It's not as if I wander around in a white coat with a stethoscope around my neck (not that they do these days). When we first moved into our house some thirty years ago, a neighbour popped round to say hello and mistook me for an Egyptian doctor. The misconception continues.

A little old lady (why are they always 'little'?) tugs at my elbow and asks me for some paracetamol for her headache. As she is hard of hearing, I have to raise my voice to explain: 'I am *not* a DOCTOR!'

In the surrounding minestrone of noise the word 'DOCTOR' catches wing. '*And once sent out – a word takes wing beyond recall.*'[14]

... and so word gets around that I am the go-to person for advice on everyone's lumbago, sciatica, dodgy hips etc. They beckon me, waving their EHICs[15] – wimmin to the left of me, wimmin to the right of me, holler and wander.[16]

Now all that remains is for one or more of the four blokes to tap lightly on my cabin door late at night with a request for Viagra.

I begin to wonder if I can deflect the misconception by informing my 'patients' that I am a solicitor, but quickly dismiss the thought. I would be inundated with requests for advice on their wills (where there's a will – there are relatives), trusts (truss?), probate, divorce settlements, boundary disputes etc. etc. Words such as 'That Perry Mason,

---

[14] Horace, *Epistles.*
[15] European Health Insurance Cards, as they were known at the time.
[16] Apologies to Tennyson.

he was such a nice man' would haunt me forever. In any event, I've given up the cut and thrust of the law. I don't get half-cut any more, and my thrust is reserved exclusively for recreation.

I'm sipping a cup of coffee, contemplating my current fate in particular and my future in general, when a woman approaches me looking ashen, not unlike someone who has just been commanded to walk the plank.

This turns out to be another 'consultation'. I listen to Jennifer's tale of woe over the loss of 'my dear Ben', who died of terminal cancer at the age of ten. She is overwrought. I try to console her in the only way I know how by mimicking my therapist: 'You have to give it time – think nice thoughts – take each day as it comes – take one step at a time' etc.

She shows me a photo of Ben taken during his last days. A flood of tears would have ensued from me, but for the fact that it transpires that Ben was a King Charles spaniel.

For pity's sake, as Gustav Holst might have said.

For dinner this evening we are served leg of lamb. The dish demonstrates perfectly how to elevate cuisine paysanne to something posh, without losing one's way in perfumed poncery. The lamb is followed by a well-constructed tarte Tartin with an apricot coulis.[17]

However, dinner is taken amongst widows crying into their soup for the loss of their loved ones. They are all, without exception, very nice. As the prevailing mood is that of 'we're all in this together', they don't hold back in sharing their sorrows. I empathise and wonder if my shoulders are broad enough to sustain a seven-day onslaught.

_____

[17] It is a relatively unknown fact that apricot stones contain cyanide.

It isn't long before my habitual solitary coffee respite break threatens to become a regular consulting session. I am determined that this is something up with which I will not put.[18] To avoid this, I think of a plan cunning enough to impress Baldrick. In a Damascene moment of revelation I decide to take coffee in my cabin. Solitary confinement was not what I had in mind when I booked the trip. Dreading solitude, I have come on the boat hoping to befriend jovial people, only to find myself surrounded by weeping women who are driving me into isolation (sob). This does not bode well for the future.

I head to the bar for Schnapps and am nonplussed by their method of measuring tots. Conversion from imperial to metric measures: arrrgh! Some things should not be measured in decimal. There are three sips to a gulp and eight gulps to a pint; what could be more simple than that?

I'm reminded of my tutor in logic and metaphysics at St Andrews, who insisted on holding his tutorial with me in the Cross Keys pub. He was invariably late and would start the tutorial by commenting on how sunny the day was (even when it wasn't) with 'Och, aye, but one swallow dunna quench a thirst.'[19] This was a cue for me to buy him a pint. Made precious little difference to his appraisal of my mediocre work, though.

... and so to bed.

---

[18] A convoluted sentence which betrays my classical 'educashun'.
[19] Very philosophical.

Day 4

We plough a rough furrow south from Rüdesheim, having left Koblenz exactly as we found it – not a cobblestone disturbed. No carousing into the early hours for us.

For dinner this evening we are presented with medallions of pressed rabbit with mushroom jus. I am not overly fond of rabbit nor of mushrooms, although all mushrooms are edible, some only once. However, this dish celebrates the onset of cooler weather. The combination of rabbit, mushrooms, butter, stock and roasted garlic is as wonderful as that first crisp day, a clear blue sky and heavy frost on the ground at the onset of winter, when leaves are falling and there's a faint smell of the first fire burning in a hearth.

At dinner I meet Agnes, who, after we have eaten, engages me in conversation. We chat idly, but before long the conversation takes a serious turn when I ask her why she has chosen this particular trip. An innocent question in normal circumstances, but, as I am soon to discover, these circumstances are far from normal.

She tells me about how she and her husband always holidayed in this part of Germany, and how much he had loved this stretch of the river. Latterly, when he could no longer walk, they had taken this boat trip every year for the last three years. She is tearful as she recounts in detail the misfortunes which befell her dear departed husband. Sadly, he died six months ago and she has come to scatter his ashes on the river. She asks if I will help her.

It's not often that I feel at a loss, but I do on this occasion. My mind races in search of a plausible excuse. I manage to convince her that this is something intensely personal and that the presence of a stranger would be inappropriate.

I wipe my tears as unobtrusively and as quickly as I can whilst preserving some degree of decorum and leave the woman alone to contemplate her sorrow.

The original diary entry relating to this ends abruptly for some reason.

Now that I think about it, I can't help feeling that I have let Agnes down badly. Not a proud moment for me. I have been put to the test and have been found wanting. This is not the shape of my heart. Under different circumstances I would have helped her; not for one moment would I have demurred. Does my moral compass need recalibrating?

This encounter is slowly unlocking the door to my chamber of horrors as images of the MND years begin to surface from the recesses of my mind. Agnes's sorry tale reduces me to tears as I recall Marilyn's tragic predicament slowly unfolding. I can see her now sitting in a darkened room in sunglasses, sorrowfully awaiting my approach to administer the next round of syringes. Her blue eyes had become hypersensitive to light, which she found painful, and so the house was shrouded in darkness even during the summer months. She had taken her last look at sunshine and brook sometime during the second year after the onset of MND. It sets me wondering why Marilyn's life had so suddenly come to that.

How loosely woven is the fabric of our happiness.

It all started following our receipt of the prognosis. Our GP placed his hand on my shoulder and levelled with me with the words, 'You need to know that this disease is not only cruel; it is brutal. You will both need to be strong,' to which my only sorrowful response was 'It should have happened to me. It should have been me.' That was the day the music died.

As the disease progressed, the only things functioning were her hearing (with two powerful hearing aids) and a brain which continued to be razor-sharp to the very end. Her eyesight was a different matter; there were times when she needed my help to see. If she wanted to watch the news and her eyelids were not responding to the messages from her brain, they would remain closed. I would stand behind her wheelchair and lift one of her eyelids between my forefinger and thumb to enable her to see. My other hand was busy sleeving tears as they rolled down my cheeks.

The trip is far from what I had contemplated and isn't helping me to heal my scars.

Repairing to the bar in my current state of mind would be a grave mistake, and so to bed with a cocktail of remorse, anxiety and grief. A sleepless night beckons.

Day 5

Another night of torment.

A rough night and a mental blur after yesterday's harrowing experience prevent my making further notes.

I dream of the day we received the diagnosis and prognosis: sitting tearfully in silence on the sofa in the garden room, staring into the middle distance, holding hands. Deep in love, with not a lot to say. I see two eyes of blue, softly whispering, 'I love you.'

Having visited all save one of the various towns previously, I eschew the excursions, which require a good deal of walking; I couldn't find any porters to carry me, not even for ready money. I am conscious of giving the impression of being standoffish or aloof, and so explain that I am here to work on the manuscript of my book. This is met with 'Am I going to be in it?'

Lunch is taken in the saloon, laid on for me and two others with mobility problems who have also remained on board. The array of buffet items is as vast and varied as the species of tree frog in the lower Congo Basin. The whole affair is displayed with rhubarb leaves the size of a punkah-wallah's fan, with spears of asparagus standing to regimental attention as if awaiting the command to 'quick march!' There are marble-smooth, knotted pouches of creamy burrata and tomatoes as pink and sweet as a mermaid's nipples (allegedly). More impressive is the quantity, variety, display and arrangement of salad leaves, which is such that I fully expect an elderly Japanese soldier to emerge from the thicket waving a white flag of surrender. All in all, technically a competent lunch, marred only by a tendency for each dish to be accompanied by a copious quantity of Liebfraumilch.

The pianist who plays in the evenings turns up and sticks to her routine, despite having an audience of only three and despite it being lunchtime. Guess what she strikes up? … 'Are You Lonesome Tonight?' I bury my head in my hands at the absurdity of it all and laugh, a laugh bordering on hysteria. I console myself with Rohinton Mistry's words from *A Fine Balance*:

> The human face has limited space … if you fill your face with laughing, there will be no more room for crying.

I remember Mr Churchill (no, not Winston), my music teacher at prep school, imploring that I listen to him carefully because, he said, he had been taught by Herbert Sumsion, who had worked with Sir Edward Elgar, who had traded tips with Sir Arthur Sullivan, who had been taught by John Goss, who in turn had studied under Thomas Attwood, who, as we all know, was one of the few English pupils of Mozart. Much good it did me.

Three physically, emotionally or psychologically impaired passengers lunching at individual well-dressed tables, listening to the lyrics of Roy Turk, is reminiscent of a Ionesco play. This, yet again, sends me off to those lonesome dark nights of song and poems.

One of the diners is the fourth man (no, he isn't the Cambridge spy), whom I have not yet met, although I have seen him here and there. He has good cheekbones and a fair tailor. He is reedy and bald, with protruding ears reminiscent of a Toby jug and an unhappy moustache. By my reckoning, he is eighty in the shade but looks younger. The sort who is inclined to push at a door marked 'Pull' and who might have scaled the dizzy heights of 'ink monitor' at his prep school. He gives the impression of one who might be an avid reader of top-shelf literature. He approaches the table reeking of camphorated oil and swaying at the knees like a rating on the bridge of a ship in a high sea, sidling up to an officer with a steaming cuppa and the words 'Cocoa, Skipper?'

I try to engage him in conversation, but his brain appears to be wired by events beyond its circuits' capacity. I now remember catching sight of him at St Pancras station as he struggled manfully with a bishop luggage trolley.[20] I catch his eye, which is met with a nod in acknowledgement, so no chance of any conversation, I think to myself.

The other diner, who sits quietly sipping her coffee, looks at me and smiles. I return the compliment and decide to engage her in conversation as a matter of courtesy. I had noticed as she approached her table that she suffered from mobility problems. She informs me that she is in the early stages of muscular dystrophy[21] and wants 'to get this trip in' whilst she can. She doesn't feel the need to elaborate because, she says, 'as a doctor, you'll understand'.

The symptoms of muscular dystrophy are something with which I have become all too familiar. I used to watch Marilyn's disease wore on and her muscles began to degenerate. As I watched Marilyn struggle, I gradually came to realise that unless she died of a heart attack or of respiratory failure, all that would remain of her former self would be the frail framework of her body – just skin and bone, with her inside it, still thinking. Her disability was

---

[20] A bishop moves diagonally in chess.

[21] Muscular dystrophy is a group of inherited genetic conditions that gradually cause the muscles to weaken, leading to increasing disability. Like MND, it is fatal.

incremental, and the gradual physical indignity was breaking her down as an individual in slow motion. Her body was becoming not unlike a building gradually falling into disrepair.

After dinner I'm sitting at the bar enveloped in sadness, nursing a particularly fine Armagnac, contemplating having survived the previous four days and girding my loins for the predictable onslaught of the next four when, yes, you might have guessed, I'm accosted by yet another passenger. She has a lazy eye, is well endowed, and smells of the cork. Without so much as a 'Comment est ton père?' she sits on a bar stool beside me. Idiot that I am, I had assumed bar stools to be a safe haven for men; not so any more.

She introduces herself as Sally (whose full name I conjure up in my mind as 'Sally Effingwell', for reasons which will soon become apparent). She sports diamanté pineapple earrings which swing like sparkling chandeliers; her clothes appear to have given her the slip, as her embonpoint places excessive strain on the buttons of her leopard print blouse. She wears trousers apparently woven from yards of drugget, as used on the backs of chairs in Victorian parsonages.

For once, this 'patient' is not seeking solace but is looking to vent her spleen. She informs me that she is on board to escape intense mental stress brought on by acrimonious divorce proceedings which are now in their fourth year. She is fighting him tooth and nail and is determined to 'take him for everything he's got, including the dog!' Given my recent experience, I don't ask about the name of the quadruped.

Contempt for him (the husband, not the dog) runs through her like veins in a Gorgonzola, as does her sulphurous and sarcastic contempt for solicitors. Though I find this irksome and am tempted to take it on a square cut, I let it go through to the wicketkeeper. 'Crikey', as Goethe wouldn't have said. 'Thank goodness I haven't let on that I'm a solicitor.'

As an afterthought, I do wonder if that is the right decision. A second opinion of her case would have been welcomed, and, with what solicitors charge these days, I could have freed my trip. Ah, well ...

After twelve years of being married to 'that oaf' she has had enough of his late-night carousing with his mates, smoking (a habit he has picked up recently) etc. This leads me to speculate as to the cause of this change in his behaviour. Is she justified, or might she have driven him to it? I am reminded of the story of a man who was pulled over by the police at three o'clock one morning for driving erratically.

Officer: 'May I ask where are you going at this time of night, sir?'

Man: 'I'm on my way to a lecture about alcohol abuse, its effect on the human body, and the evils of gambling and carousing all night.'

Officer: 'Oh, really? And who is giving the lecture at this late hour?'

Man: 'That would be my wife.'

Could Sally be the architect of her own misfortune? Clucking and becoming more bitter each time she mentions lawyers, she scatters vituperative epithets like confetti. Her discourse is interminable. Bindweed starts growing around my ankles; a caterpillar completes its life cycle and flies out through an open window.

She expects me to be more sympathetic than I am. 'Disappointing, given your profession', she exclaims. If it was a cry for help, I didn't want to hear it.

Anything I say seems incomprehensible to her ears, and not just because she appears to have done nothing about tgeir wax build-up. When I try to suggest a possible solution to her problems, she gets the sort of look on her face that you see in dogs when you show them a card trick. Her brain seems incapable of receiving information from the outside. I do, however, learn some interesting new words. I can't swear they are from Beowulf, but they definitely sound Anglo-Saxon.

Her sole purpose in life is to serve as a warning to others. I'm fully aware that married life doesn't suit everyone. Indeed, a twice-divorced friend of mine explained why he was resolute in his determination to avoid getting married again: 'If you lock up your wife and your dog in separate rooms for a couple of hours, when you open their doors, which of them is pleased to see you?' Ouch!

Sally announces that she's off to the back of the boat, where she might find a more sympathetic ear. I'm tempted to correct her with 'it's called the *stern*' but think better of it in the circumstances. There's a special place in hell reserved for pedants like me.

It transpires that I am not the only victim of her tirade. I witness other passengers who, having received a full blast of her venom, give her a wide berth. She belongs in purgatory, for without her it would not be purgatory.

Is there no one to whom I can turn for solace? Quis consolatur ipsos consolatores?[22]

I am desperate to escape this oppressive atmosphere which gives me such grief and deprives me of the respite I so

---

[22] 'Who will console the consoler?' Apologies to the Roman poet Juvenal for borrowing from his *Satires*: 'Quis custodiet ipsos custodes?' – 'Who will guard the guards?'

desperately crave. Should I jump ship and hitchhike to the nearest port? It would be easy-peasy[23] in a river; just swim to the other bank, a quick change of clothes, leave my old persona behind, and Robert est ton oncle. After all, if old Johnny Stonehouse can do it, why not me?

To the bar once more; I order a double Phyllosan[24] on the rocks. By now, dear reader, you will have noticed the insidious influence of my fellow passengers through the ever-so-subtle change in my post-prandial tipple from alcohol to tinctures of their supposedly health-giving properties.

And ... so to bed.

I feel something inside me is dying. What that something is, I am unable to say or think or feel. I only know that I feel terribly alone in the world now. Never again will I see Marilyn seated at the piano playing, or smiling at me across the table as she triumphally lays down her cards with the hand that so often beat me.

With these many thoughts, contrary to my expectations, I fall into a deep sleep.

---

[23] A Japanese colloquialism.

[24] 'Phyllosan Fortifies the Over-40s' (1960). Calcium phosphate, icing sugar, starch, powdered acacia, talc, magnesium stearate, sucrose, calcium carbonate, gum sandarac substitute, wax, titanium dioxide (E171) and colouring (E153). Now available in liquid form.

Day 6

This morning's excursion is to Heidelberg, the one excursion I join. This involves a journey by coach. Each passenger boards the coach clutching a packed lunch, except one, who ascends the steps with a holdall and, catching my eye, deposits her not incredible bulk beside me with the look of one who has lost a twenty-pound note and found a fiver. It transpires that the holdall is laden with victuals: breadsticks, cheddar cheese, Ritz crackers etc. She proceeds to feast on the journey to the sound of popping Tupperware like a volley of starting pistols.

Being seated at such close proximity, I can't help but notice her sartorial inelegance. She has brought with her a cushion which she places at the small of her back for support. Nothing wrong in that, of course, but the cushion looks familiar; somewhere there is an old Ford Cortina missing its cushion covers. She is wearing elasticated trousers of the type worn by women who order from the back covers of magazines. She seems to be in permanent state of dishabille, giving the impression that her chest has fallen into her drawers.

She spends some time telling me her life story. Angelina hails from Zimbabwe, (Southern Rhodesia to old Africa hands). No one else has worked such vigour into the name 'Zimbabwe'. She makes its two Bs slap against each other like rubberised domination paddles (allegedly). Her late father was a Dutch tobacco farmer in Zimbabwe; she was born to his Chinese mistress. Her late husband, a pied-noir who had emigrated to southern Africa from Algeria, had made his fortune in the manufacture of urinal cakes. She speaks with a guttural accent and with a mild ululation when she talks of her husband's demise. She appears to be three minorities all rolled into one.

She is sporting an ever-so-thin black moustache and wisps of a beard. Had I courage enough, I would be able to count the number of individual hairs that descend from her bottom lip. If you don't want to listen to what people are saying and are captive in their presence, it is not unnatural to concentrate on their features and draw caricatures in your mind.

The 'consultation' lasts a lifetime, for she doesn't stop to draw breath. The Gregorian chant 'Missa de Angelis' is comfortably shorter. Roger Bannister could have run almost the length of London's Piccadilly and still have had time to pop into Fortnum & Mason to order his Christmas hamper.

Notwithstanding that Angelina has a problem with mobility, at the sound of the dinner gong, she moves faster than a mobility scooter hurtling towards Greggs at closing time.

The nosebag this evening is king prawns in garlic. Though plump and juicy in their own right, they are not exactly majestic in size – more Prince Edward prawns than King Charles.

For Mains, a casserole of an ingenious fusion of tastes, perfectly balanced so that the herbs do not overwhelm the spicy saucisson or vice versa.

Another challenging dinner, to which I'm becoming mildly inured. The main problem is that dining places are not allocated and therefore I have no say in who sits at the same table as me.

Dinner is taken with the usual interruptions. I am joined by Joan, who slurps her soup with the aid of a straw. I recognise this as possibly dysphagia,[25] one of the conditions from which Marilyn suffered severely. I suffer a tsunami of emotions – including sympathy for Joan, but also, more disturbingly, anguish at being reminded of Marilyn's suffering. I find myself thinking of the time when, following her PEG surgery, she awoke in the early hours of the morning in great pain, which had to be relieved by my performing a 'procedure' on her stomach as guided by a consultant nurse on a phone.

I listen to the conversation at the table with closed ears and closed mind. I try to daydream through the meal, but to no avail. I wolf down my casserole and beat a hasty retreat with a mind improving book to what I misguidedly think to be the relative sanctuary of a corner of the bar.

What, dear reader, do you suppose happens next?

After some time I look up and see no one. Not a soul; 'Mein Gott!' as Günter Grass would have said. The saloon is empty. I begin to wonder if I have missed an announcement; have the passengers been called to muster stations?

I enquire of a steward who has been busy tidying the shelves under the bar counter and has therefore been out of sight. He tells me that the saloon usually empties at about nine thirty every evening, almost as if a factory hooter has sounded the end of a shift. Apparently passengers descend to their cabins at that time of night to take their medication, recalibrate their pacemakers, partake of blood transfusions, receive heart transplants etc. and, whilst there, they

---

[25] A condition which makes it difficult to swallow certain foods or drinks, and in its severe form leaves the sufferer unable to swallow at all. Signs of dysphagia include coughing or choking when eating or drinking, or bringing food back up, sometimes through the nose.

generally decide to turn in rather than enquire of the energy
to go back upstairs. It occurs to me that *that's* what must
have happened to the *Mary Celeste*; it's just that those who
discovered her failed to look below deck.

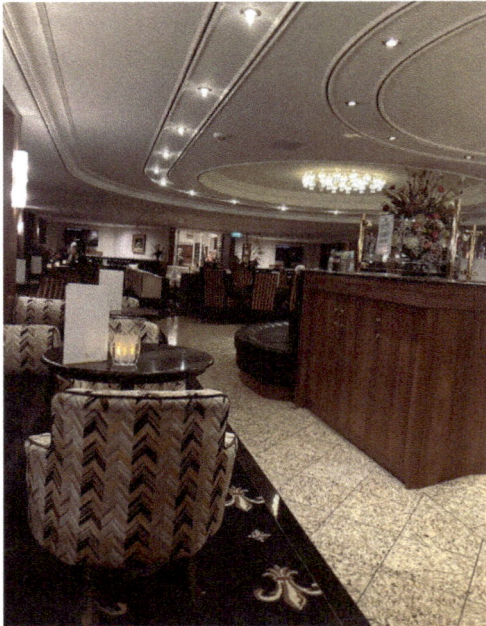

The deserted saloon, 9.25 pm

It is here, in more sombre moments, that I get a glimpse of
my future. I see my fellow travellers shuffling instead of
walking, leaning instead of standing, moving with the aid of
walking sticks, standing in doorways etc. Are we not all
wondering if or when we might meet one of the present-day
Four Horsemen of the Apocalypse: heart disease, cancer,
neurogenerative disease and metabolic dysfunction? And,
before that, we face the prospect of the other Big Four:
dementia, disability, divorce and debt. A great majority of us

have been afflicted at some stage by one or more, to which we can now add the inescapable death and taxes.

I am sitting in the saloon, a glass of Armagnac in hand, when my mind wanders in a direction I have assiduously sought to avoid. I see Marilyn sitting in silence, motionless, gazing at her lap, her head bowed. I am numbed by the image. There were times when the stillness and the silence forced me to see if she was still alive.

I shake myself out of the emotional trance and set my glass down with trembling hand to wipe away my tears. I begin to wonder what has triggered the image. After all, there is no weeping widow sitting beside me. For once I have been left alone.

It doesn't take me long to realise that the trigger is *silence*. It is silence that haunts me; it is the silence I am seeking to escape that drove me to this boat in the first place, and yet, and yet, I am confronted with it again. Small wonder that tears well up inside me.

I swap my Armagnac for something stronger: a Sanatogen[26] martini, not shaken, not stirred, but whisked. 'Bugger the ice; I need a stiff one tonight,' I say to the bartender.

And so to bed.

---

[26] Sanatogen: a tonic wine introduced some fifty years ago, made by the traditional blending of full-bodied ruby British wine with the special Sanatogen formula to produce the unique mellow flavour. I believe it was also available 'with added iron'.

Day 7

I wake up sobbing. I have been dreaming about Marilyn
sitting in her wheelchair, head bowed, and I'm seized with a
panic that the moment I have so dreaded and which I have
pushed to the back of my mind has finally arrived. The
muscles in her neck have collapsed: not unexpected, but
nevertheless agonising to watch. The importance of neck
muscles should not be underestimated. Lacking the support
of her muscles, her head flops this way and that as a rag
doll's head. The time has come to apply the neck brace, and I
hit a psychological wall which I find difficult to overcome. I
struggle to see how I can attach the neck brace without
physically lifting her head, which means that both of my
hands will be occupied. I don't know whether it will be
painful for her or whether she wants it. I feel acutely
distressed as I fumble with the straps. I am struggling to see
what I am doing; my eyesight is obscured by tears.

The day passes uneventfully as 'they' are on an extended
excursion.

The captain's dinner tonight. I decline her invitation to dine
at her table on the not unreasonable grounds that one
draws the line at dining with a member of the crew.

The obsession that the navy has with rank knows no bounds.
I'm reminded of a conversation said to have taken place in
one of London's military clubs amongst the three service
chiefs when the rank of field marshal was abolished
(presumably because the army had run out of fields to
marshal). The head of the Royal Navy was pleased to have
retained his title of First Sea Lord. The head of the Royal Air
Force, Air Chief Marshal, being unhappy with his title (which
he said sounded too French), wondered if he might not be

COPING WITH GRIEF AND EXORCISING DEMONS

granted the title of 'First Air Lord'. The head of the army, a general, protested at being called the First Land Lord ... but I digress.

I must face the consequences of eschewing hoi oligoi and choosing to consort with hoi polloi, for I notice that, dressed to the nines as they are, the men are wont to discard their coats[27] and drape them over their chairs without so much as an enquiring nod for consent from those present at their table. I discard my coat on only two occasions: when I am playing a sport, out of convenience, and when making love, as a matter of courtesy.

Tonight's culinary delight for our farewell repast is chicken cacciatore. I partake of the chicken cacciatore, which involves a chewy hunk of white bird like a flexed bicep. They say it was free-range, which of course is a good thing, but I fear this bird, what with the low-security nature of its incarceration, was allowed to slip out too regularly to the gym in the village. The rich tomatoey sauce and pasta would have made it a cosy and nurturing dish on a cold April night had it been served with anything other than a bicep.

I am joined at dinner by Amanda, an elderly spinster, straight of spine and wearing tweed. Her posture belies her background. She has been rather unfortunate in her choice of ancestors and is possessed of a remarkable absence of intellectual endowment. I get the impression that she is a relict. I notice that the fine merino wool cardigan she so nonchalantly tosses over the back of her chair is so moth-eaten it resembles a woolly colander.

When one spends time in close proximity to someone, one notices their eating habits and very quickly one is apt to find

---

[27] The correct term is 'coats', not 'jackets'; only potatoes wear jackets.

oneself concentrating on their quirks. Sitting opposite, I
begin to notice the way she chews her meat, not unlike a
cow chewing the cud; her jaw is moving sideways as
opposed to up and down. Until now I have not been aware
of the different ways in which people chew their food. Her
manner of chewing requires her jaw to undergo remarkable
oral gymnastics.

She notices me watching her method of chewing, and
explains that she has come on the trip to convalesce from
the reconstruction of her jaw following cancer treatment
and is praying for remission. 'But, as a doctor, you will know
all about it,' she chirps. *Here we go again*, I muse.

Dinner is followed by a quiz of mind-numbing banality and
a dinner dance. With Wincarnis[28] flowing liberally over
dinner, the passengers are getting feisty. Over-vigorous
'hands in the air' dancing action looks likely to do serious
damage to their rotator cuffs and expose unsightly wet
patches under the arms like one of those old Sure
deodorant ads. Will we be privy to an 'incident' on the dance
floor, I wonder?

Having resolved to get into the spirit of things, I espy a
likely (a term I use loosely) dance partner for a possible
paso doble, and so a lawyer's primeval instinct to conduct
due diligence kicks in. After circumnavigating her frame. I
come to the inescapable conclusion that this is not for me.
Good call, as the dancing involves passengers forming a

---

[28] Wincarnis Original Tonic Wine: a blend of enriched wine and malt
extract infused with a bewildering variety of botanicals. A popular drink
particularly amongst women 'of a certain age', who swore by its health-
giving properties (as if) and who drank it surreptitiously straight from
the bottle, which was usually secreted in the larder behind a bag of self-
rising flour.

circle, raising and lowering their arms and occasionally stamping their feet. Having noticed me circumventing her girth, she approaches me between dances and, fearing that any eye contact might be met with requisitions on title and a request for further and better particulars, I resolve to avoid looking her way in the way a pig is wont to avoid the butcher's eye.

Unexpectedly I witness what turns out to be the highlight of the evening. I am thrilled to catch a glimpse of an ankle, albeit encased in a surgical stocking. The whole affair smacks of *Hi-de-Hi*!

It doesn't take long for me to realise that survival is a matter not of taking part but of observing. This pays dividends when I see one of the male passengers approaching the dancefloor, portentously escorting a waddling woman who is rubbing her hips with an expression of 'look, no Zimmer!'

Ay oop, I think. *There goes a classic case of two hips and no hooray!*

Just before midnight, purely by chance (methinks), I run into a not uncomely female member of the crew, Charlotta (for that is her name, she assures me), in the coffee lounge. I have wandered in for some cocoa, as one does, just before turning in. The two of us being the only ones present, we chat about this and that for a while, and, being the dunce that I am, it takes me a while to wonder – am I being propositioned?

If I am, what is the honourable thing to do?

If I'm not, but I mistakenly think that I am, will she raise the alarm? Will I find myself unceremoniously in the presence of a burly member of the Bundespolizei, who I'm told are not

averse to breaking heads? They too don't eat Marmite.
British police, on the other hand, eat a tad too much of it, I
suspect.

Mild panic sets in. Various scenarios play out in my mind at
lightning speed.

Is it true that you never forget to ride a bicycle?

How many frogs (to my one) has she kissed?

How does something like this work? What are the rules?
What is the etiquette?

Will declining the invitation constitute 'scorn'? What *exactly*
is a woman scorned?

Will my refusal be met with a glare at breakfast? Will my
declining the invitation result in her accidently spilling hot
coffee in my lap?

Will I be met at breakfast with either mild derision or
applause by some of her colleagues, who may have placed
bets on the outcome?

Is paranoia setting in?

This is my opportunity to deploy the silk dressing gown,
surely? On the other hand, is it best to leave it unmolested
on its hanger?

Isn't this why I am here?

Suddenly I remember that my therapist is expecting to be
debriefed.

... but then so am I?

Carpe noctem! But then, on the other hand ...

... and the denouement?

Did she or didn't she? Did I or didn't I? Did we or didn't we?

Is the answer buried within the narrative? Or it is not?

The diary entry ends abruptly here.

Well may you speculate. I leave you, dear reader, to work it out. There's a limit to how much entertainment I can provide at my expense.

Suffice it to say that what happens on the boat stays on the boat.

The various tales of woe play tricks on my brain; the dreams return in my sleep uninvited. It's a little after three, and my head is resting on a soaking pillow again. I am deprived of the sweet sleep of the innocent. I am visited in my bed by an episode which emotionally cleaves me in two.

The uncharacteristic movement of Amanda's jaw I witnessed during dinner leads me to relive a nightmare incident towards the end of Marilyn's life. It is one of those moments when I go close to Marilyn to see if she is still breathing and notice blood dripping from a corner of her mouth. Holding her chin up, I try to open her mouth, only to discover that her jaw has locked tight. Try as I might, I cannot release it. With trembling hands I dial for help, and after what seems an interminable interval I finally receive the advice that the only way to release a locked jaw, other than surgery, is for the patient to relax, or to inject a muscle relaxant. No force from without will unlock a jaw. Medical intervention is not an option as I have neither the skill nor the resources to bring about the desired result. Syringes I have aplenty, but not the necessary medication.

With faltering voice I am explaining the situation to Marilyn, knowing she is hoping against hope that paramedics are at the door. 'I'm so sorry Mel, it's only you and me – only you and me, Mel – there's no one else here. We will get over this together, just as we have the other obstacles in the past. Remember in the beginning? We agreed that together we would tackle whatever it throws at us. Stay strong.'

The jaw is firmly locked , and I whisper softly to her that it may release if she can relax. I'm kneeling beside Marilyn, holding her knuckles with one hand (the finger braces having tried to do their best, her fingers have curled into her wrists), and with the other I massage her jaw. Beads of fear run down my face. I can think of nothing to help her relax, so I sing 'Morningtown Ride', the lullaby I used to sing to my children.

I watch the digital clock by her side, for the medics may want to know how long it is taking. It takes a long forty-two minutes.

When the locked jaw is released, I discover to my horror and distress that it has bitten her tongue in four places. As I clean the lesions on her tongue and apply a painkilling gel to them, I sense the tension release in her body. I tuck the blanket under her chin, gently kiss her forehead and tiptoe away. I can feel her body leaking sadness and her mind in deep sorrow.

I drag myself to the bedroom with leaden feet, limp arms hanging by my side. With aching heart, I grab a box of tissues and fall onto my bed. I curl up in a ball and I cry – the crying of the inconsolable – and yet again, as all too often, I bury my head deep into my pillow lest she should hear me crying.

I vowed then that mine would be the last face that Marilyn saw ... and so it was.

Day 8

We have stopped; the jolt of the boat mooring awakens me. We have arrived at our final destination of Cologne. I lie awake in bed at a time when problems, woes and worries loom large. The thoughts and images that visit when one is in a sleepless trance cannot be easily dismissed.

I force myself out of bed, slip some clothes on and, as I am heading for the promenade deck, quite by chance, I come across someone I knew well a few years ago. He doesn't shake my hand or crack a smile. He used to be a good friend. I struggle to recognise the face – gaunt, haggard, dishevelled and drawn, with shallow cheeks and bloodshot eyes. 'There's a face that tells a story of suffering – of having been through the wars and walked on hot coals,' I mutter as I tear myself away from the mirror.

Together Marilyn and I fought many battles, all the while knowing that the war was lost. The essential thing, I kept telling myself, was to have fought well.

After breakfast I thank and say goodbye to some of the crew. One particular member of the crew thanks me for the enjoyable 'chit-chat'[29] last night, and I echo her sentiment.

As I board the coach to the Gare du Nord, I breathe a sigh of relief; the nightmare is finally over. My fellow passengers gaze out of the window in silence, deep in thought about what awaits them. I am reliably informed that normally the coach would ring with the chatter of its occupants. There is no one sitting in the seat next to mine; the empty chair syndrome kicks in again. Back to the future?

---

[29] Chit-chat: an interesting turn of phrase. I make a mental note for its possible use in the future!

As the coach stops at some traffic lights, looking out of the window, I see a young couple strolling, smiling, holding hands. It brings a smile to my lips. What is it that makes me smile? The fact that he has just stolen a kiss, or that they are holding hands?

I have always felt that holding hands is the single most powerful subliminal emotion two people can exchange in silence, in sorrow, in pain, in love, in sympathy, in consolation, in happiness etc. It is a physical act which transcends all in the meaning it conveys in absolute silence. One only holds hands with someone intimately close, be it helping an aged parent across a road or stopping to admire a beautiful sunset with someone you love. However good and close a friend may be, holding their hand even in those circumstances would be taboo.

It begins with a baby clutching the little finger of a parent at birth and ends with them holding someone's hand at the time of their death.

Take the example of the Boeing 747 flight BA009 from Heathrow to New Zealand, with 263 occupants on board, on 24 June 1982. When in midair, all four engines failed and the plane descended rapidly. As the pilot signalled 'mayday' and oxygen masks dropped on the passengers, according to those present there was no hysteria. A passenger commented, 'Mothers moved to comfort their children; husbands reached for their wives' hands.'

When the time came there could be no conversation with Marilyn and, although she had no hands as such, my holding her knuckles in silence was all that was needed.

When I die, I wish to die with someone holding my hand, whatever the circumstances.

The sight of that couple leads me to thinking nice thoughts: something I encouraged Marilyn to do to avoid being maudlin. I was lucky to have been with her for more than fifty years, and we too held hands and smiled at each other.

The thought produces euphoria, which vanishes faster than a gambler's lucky streak as I remember hugging Marilyn tightly following an incident. That memory leads me to relive the moment when she tried to hug me with what little strength she had left, to put her weak and failing arms around me for what, although I wasn't to know at the time, was effectively to be the last time. It was then that I understood, irrespective of physical strength, how strongly the body can feel love for someone.

I settle down in the car taking me home. I find it difficult to relax. It doesn't help that the 'driver' has the loosest possible relationship with whatever lane he is supposed to be in. I have time enough to reflect on the past and on the present and realise with foreboding what the future holds for me. I am tired of chewing on the gristle of life.

Having endured nigh on three years of horror, my attempt at exorcising the demons which haunt me relentlessly has proved to be an abject failure.

Damn MND – for inflicting physical, emotional and psychological torture on Marilyn for three years; for draining the life out of her by the minute.

Damn MND again – for driving me to the very brink as I tended to Marilyn's needs and watched her uncomplainingly die ever so slowly, in sorrow and in pain, as each muscle in her body ceased to function and gradually wasted away.

Damn Brexit – for depriving me of much-needed domiciliary care to help me in my earnest endeavours to support Marilyn.

And damn COVID – for depriving Marilyn of the medical attention she so desperately needed, and for depriving me of the clinical support I craved.

Circumstances conspired to make our lives a living hell on a daily basis. On two separate occasions that I can recall, over a period of three years, the margin between my 'tipping over' and retaining my sanity was as thin as cigarette paper. MND destroyed Marilyn, and it came within a whisker of destroying me as I fought against all odds to care for her.

> *Every person is responsible for all the good within the scope of his abilities and no more, and none can tell whose sphere is the largest.*[30]

There are times when I can feel the forces of hell which were unleashed upon Marilyn and which finally overwhelmed her.

This boat trip has managed to condense into eight days the harrowing nightmare which Marilyn and I endured for three years.

At the Gare du Nord, I struggle to read the departure board through misty eyes and curse, for no amount of rubbing them seems to make a difference – a simple enough movement of which Marilyn was deprived. My effort to read the board sends me into a spin of painful reminiscence of the first occasion I helped Marilyn to watch the news by holding her eyelids open, when something touched me deep inside.

There are moments when I feel overwhelmed by a sense of deep loss, and at such times I am set to wondering what moment in our past I will continue to miss the most in the future. I have come to dread the golden autumn days we so enjoyed, which lie ahead.

[30] Gail Hamilton, essayist, 1862.

DENOUEMENT

We read fine things, but never feel them to the full, until we have gone the same steps as the author.

John Keats[31]

From the car taking me home I give my therapist, April Winters, a full debriefing, as promised. She tells me that it's OK for me to feel sorry for myself.

'That's all very well,' I say, 'but will it replace the bicycle?' It's all about cycology, innit?

My therapist is now in therapy.

A sense of humour is essential; it's not funny not having one.

It is my fault, of course, for taking this trip. On reflection it doesn't take Columbo, Jessica Fletcher, Hercule Poirot, Miss Marple and the occupants of 221B Baker Street to work out that such a trip would be wholly unpredictable, and that its success or otherwise depended on pure luck.

And the outcome?

Despite the sorrow which I had locked away surfacing, I have avoided emotional anarchy. Only on one occasion on

---

[31] Letter to John Hamilton Reynolds (1818).

the boat did I come close to total despair, but I didn't 'tip over'; I managed to retain my sanity.

Those whom the gods would destroy, they first make mad.

They say that the first sign of madness is when you repeat yourself.

They say that the first sign of madness is when you repeat yourself.

In the taxi I feel my world spinning off its axis. I am anxious about the emptiness and the infernal silence which awaits me at my destination. As the car winds its way through London, emotional storms begin to gather and ever so slowly, overcome with emotion, uninvited, tears begin to flow freely, for I know it's not over. I feel a bad moon on the rise.

The silence of which I speak is all too pervasive and defies definition. It is akin to that of a seashore village when the Vikings have just departed. The thought of entering an empty house (it's not a home) continues to fill me with dread. I get the feeling that my future is in the past.

When I arrive at the front door I cannot bring myself to turn the key. I linger for some moments, reluctant to open the door I avoid the inevitable silence waiting to greet me by walking around the garden, ostensibly to see if the shrubs have suffered in my absence.

Eventually, I brace myself. As I am turning the key, the door swings open and I'm greeted by my housekeeper Olena with a smile and the words, 'Good, you have come; I will make tea.'   I am surprised to see her because I had asked her to come the following day, rather than today, as I was not sure of the time of my arrival. I am overwhelmed by her act of kindness and thoughtfulness – a sensation I have not experienced for nigh on five years.

But, of course, it's not over till it's over.

When in *Paradise Lost* Milton's Satan stood in the pit of hell and raged at heaven, he was merely a trifle miffed compared to how I feel. I am and will forever be haunted by an image that fills me with deep anguish, and which time and time again I see in my mind when faced with the sort of silence of which I speak. It is that of a single moment one night when, kneeling beside Marilyn and stroking her hair, trying to comfort her, I catch, wholly unexpectedly, sight of a tear emerging from the corner of one eye and ever so slowly roll down her cheek. It is the most profound speechless expression of her sorrow, torment and pain that I was ever to witness. Had I the prescience to realise that at the time, I would have captured that tear and stored it in a phial for the rest of my life.

In that moment – that solitary moment – the single teardrop encapsulated three years of sorrow, of pain and of suffering. It is an image that will never leave me. That tear summed up our circumstances and situation in a nutshell. It conveyed a greater meaning for me than the river of tears I had cried.

There isn't a day that goes by when I don't hear myself whispering, 'It should have been *me* … it should have been *me*.'

… and what of tomorrow?

I pray each night for my world to be restored to its axis.

EPILOGUE

My bit part in this tragic story was brought home to me by two very close friends whom Marilyn and I had known since our student days. They cared very deeply for both Marilyn and me, and came down from Aberdeen before we went into quarantine to see Marilyn 'for the last time'.

They kept in constant touch with me by phone throughout the MND years and came to know and understand my wrestling in detail.

Some months after Marilyn died, they sent me what they termed a framed 'tribute', with an inscription (*see image overleaf*).

TO MANZOOR

If you looked in the mirror - what would you see
A face full of anger and hypocrisy

Would you study the eyes with their bridge to the soul
and say – there's a person whose honesty shows

Would the lines tell some story
Of trouble you knew
And how you had struggled
To finally pull through

Would the features combined say - there's someone who's kind
With benevolent heart
For the rest of mankind

Charles M Moore

WITH DEEP RESPECT FOR YOUR FORTITUDE, DEVOTION AND STOICISM

Fiona & Anthony Summerfield
January 2015

To Manzoor
With Our Deep Respect For
Your Fortitude, Devotion and Stoicism

If you looked in the mirror – what would you see
A face full of anger and hypocrisy

Would you study the eyes with their bridge to the soul
And say – there's a person whose honesty shows

Would the lines tell some story
Of trouble you knew

And how you had struggled
To finally pull through

Would the features combined say – there's someone
who's kind
With benevolent heart
For the rest of mankind

Charles M Moore